Basic Guide to Dental Procedures

BASIC GUIDE TO DENTAL PROCEDURES

Carole Hollins

BDS
General Dental Practitioner
Member of the Panel of Examiners
National Examining Board for Dental Nurses

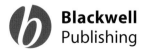 **Blackwell** Publishing

This edition first published 2008
© 2008 Carole Hollins

Blackwell Munksgaard, formerly an imprint of Blackwell Publishing was acquired by John Wiley & Sons in February 2007. Blackwell's publishing programme has been merged with Wiley's global Scientific, Technical, and Medical business to form Wiley-Blackwell.

Registered office
John Wiley & Sons Ltd, The Atrium, Southern Gate, Chichester,
West Sussex, PO19 8SQ, United Kingdom

Editorial office
9600 Garsington Road, Oxford, OX4 2DQ, United Kingdom

For details of our global editorial offices, for customer services and for information about how to apply for permission to reuse the copyright material in this book please see our website at www.wiley.com/wiley-blackwell.

The right of the author to be identified as the author of this work has been asserted in accordance with the Copyright, Designs and Patents Act 1988.

Library of Congress Cataloging-in-Publication Data

Hollins, Carole.
Basic guide to dental procedures / Carole Hollins.
p. ; cm.
Includes bibliographical references and index.
ISBN-13: 978-1-4051-5397-3 (pbk. : alk. paper)
1. Dentistry–Handbooks, manuals, etc. I. Title.
[DNLM: 1. Dentistry–methods–Handbooks. WU 49 H741b 2008]

RK56.H65 2008
617.6–dc22
2007042411

A catalogue record for this book is available from the British Library.

Set in 10 on 12.5 pt Sabon by SNP Best-set Typesetter Ltd, Hong Kong
Printed in Singapore by C. O. S. Printers Pte Ltd

1 2008

CONTENTS

*This one's for Tony – a true English gentleman –
and his darling little friend BG.*

ACKNOWLEDGEMENTS

Sincere thanks, and grateful relief, to my sister Sue for her extensive knowledge of both computers and digital cameras – thank goodness for that!

Also to the many patients who have been only too pleased to pose at various stages of their dental treatment whilst I've taken the necessary photographs to compile the book.

And, finally, to Katrina and Amy at Blackwell Publishing for their unstinting help, support and enthusiasm for the end product.

HOW TO USE THIS BOOK

As the title suggests, the book has been written as an introductory guide to the more usual dental procedures carried out in a modern dental practice. It does not attempt to explain the full theoretical and clinical technique behind these procedures; rather, it aims to give a sufficient overview, with the use of 'before and after' colour photographs, to hopefully make the book useful in helping to explain certain dental procedures to patients.

However, the main readership is envisaged to be dental care professionals, especially those unqualified or inexperienced dental nurses who may not have access to the viewing of many of the procedures described, as many practices begin to specialise in providing dental care only in certain areas of dentistry. It should be used, then, in conjunction with the excellent textbooks already available for dental nurse training, where more detail of the instruments used and other underpinning knowledge is provided.

The text in each section is laid out to explain the reasons behind the treatment described, the relevant dental background, the basics of how each procedure is carried out, and any aftercare information necessary. It is beyond the remit of the book to cover every current technique in every dental discipline discussed, and so it is hoped that the text provides at least the basic information required for the reader to gain an understanding of the procedure, before seeking a greater depth of knowledge elsewhere.

Wherever possible, the correct dental terminology has been adhered to; however, as the dental knowledge of the expected readership will vary widely, a glossary of terms has been included to clarify certain definitions in the context to which they have been referred in the text.

SECTION 1
PREVENTIVE TECHNIQUES

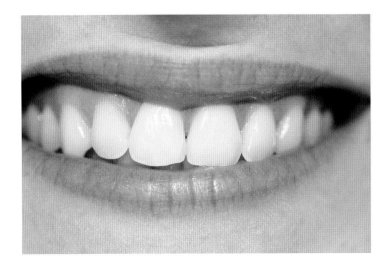

REASON FOR PROCEDURE

Preventive techniques are aimed at preventing the onset of dental caries in teeth, so that they maintain the dental health of a patient.

The two procedures to be discussed are:

• Application of fissure sealants

• Application of topical fluorides

APPLICATION OF FISSURE SEALANTS

Background information of procedure

Any surface area of a tooth that cannot be cleaned easily by the patient can allow food debris and, ultimately, plaque to accumulate there, and can allow caries to develop by acting as a stagnation area.

The usual sites are the occlusal pits and fissures of posterior teeth, and especially the first permanent molars which erupt at around 6 years of age.

These teeth are particularly prone to caries because:

• They are the least accessible teeth for cleaning, being at the back of a young patient's mouth

• They erupt at an age when a good oral hygiene regime is unlikely to have been developed, and so may be cleaned poorly

• Younger patients often have a diet containing more sugars than an adult diet, as the concept of dietary control will not be appreciated

Details of procedure

The occlusal pit or fissure needs to be eliminated to prevent it acting as a stagnation area, and this is achieved by closing the inaccessible depths with a sealant material.

The materials used are either composites or glass ionomer cements, or a combination of the two (known as a compomer).

Technique

- The tooth is kept isolated from saliva contamination, as materials will not adhere to the tooth

- Occlusal fissures and pits are chemically roughened with acid etch to allow microscopic bonding of the material to the enamel

- Etch is washed off and the tooth is dried; the etched surface will appear chalky white

- Unfilled resin is run into the etched areas to seal the fissures or pits, and then locked into the enamel structure by setting with a curing lamp

APPLICATION OF TOPICAL FLUORIDES

Background information of procedure

Other areas of the teeth which are very difficult to clean are the points at which they contact with each other in the dental arch – the interproximal (interdental) areas.

There are certain oral health products available specifically for the cleaning of these areas, such as dental floss, but they require a certain amount of dexterity and determination by the patient to be used effectively.

All fluoridated toothpastes provide some protection of these areas from caries, but some patients require additional fluoride protection by the application of topical fluoride.

They are:

- Children with high caries rates

- Disabled patients who are unable to achieve a good level of oral hygiene

- Medically compromised patients in whom tooth extractions are too dangerous to be carried out (haemophiliacs, those suffering from some heart defects)

Details of procedure

A high concentration of fluoride is required to be applied to the interproximal areas; it should be sufficiently viscous so that it is not washed away quickly by saliva and can be taken into the enamel structure of the tooth to make it more resistant to caries.

Technique

- The teeth are polished to remove any plaque present and to allow maximum tooth contact with the fluoride

- Polish is washed off thoroughly and the teeth are dried

- Viscous fluoride gel is placed into a special applicator tray (one for each arch) and the trays are inserted into the patient's mouth to fully cover the teeth

- The trays are kept *in situ* for several minutes to allow the maximum penetration of the gel into the interproximal areas

- The trays are removed and the patient is instructed not to rinse his or her teeth, or to eat or drink for up to 1 h

SECTION 2
ORAL HYGIENE INSTRUCTION

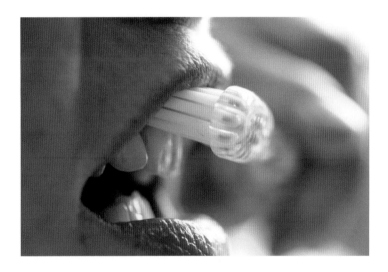

REASON FOR PROCEDURE

Oral hygiene instruction is given to patients to ensure that they are maximising their efforts to remove plaque from their teeth in order to minimise the damage caused by periodontal disease and caries.

Dietary advice is also given to help patients to avoid foods and drinks that are particularly damaging to their teeth – those high in refined sugars and those that are acidic.

When the advice is correctly followed on a regular basis, patients can enjoy a well cared for and pain-free mouth, as well as avoiding the expense of reparative dental treatment.

The procedures to be discussed are:

- Use of disclosing agents

- Toothbrushing

- Interdental cleaning

USE OF DISCLOSING AGENTS

Background information of procedure

Disclosing agents are vegetable dyes supplied in liquid or tablet form and in various colours, usually red or blue.

They act by staining any plaque on the tooth surface to their own colour, thus making it far easier to show the presence and location of the plaque to the patient, as plaque is normally a creamy white colour and may be difficult to see otherwise (see **Figure 2.1a, b**).

Once stained, suitable oral hygiene instruction can be given to remove the plaque effectively. The dyes do not stain the teeth themselves, or any restorations.

ORAL HYGIENE INSTRUCTION

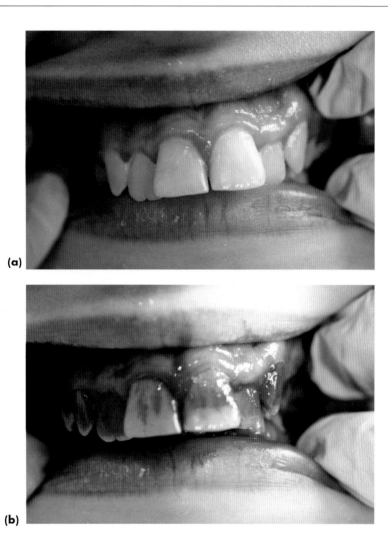

(a)

(b)

Figure 2.1 (a) Plaque on teeth. (b) Same teeth after disclosing to show plaque more obviously

Details of procedure

The agents can initially be used at the practice by the oral health team, so that the correct problem areas can be identified and suitable cleaning advice given. The patient can then use the agents at home to check his or her progress on a regular basis. The most common agents are disclosing tablets.

Technique

- A protective bib is placed over the patient so that his or her clothing is not inadvertently marked

- The patient is given one disclosing tablet and asked to chew it for about 1 min

- The patient spits out the chewed tablet and saliva, but does not rinse out

- Using a patient mirror, any stained plaque is pointed out by the oral health team and the worst areas are noted (very often the gingival margins)

- Detailed advice is then given on improved brushing techniques to eliminate the plaque from these areas

- The patient can follow these instructions immediately, so that all the stained plaque is removed, under the supervision of the oral health team

- With the plaque easily visible as a result of the disclosing agent, the patient is able to see his or her own progress and to develop the skill to maintain good oral hygiene

TOOTHBRUSHING

Background information of procedure

Toothbrushing is the most common method used to remove plaque from the easily accessible flat surfaces of the teeth, but not from the interdental areas (see **Figure 2.2**).

Many toothbrushing techniques have been suggested over the years – especially side-to-side brushing and rotary brushing – but the technique used

ORAL HYGIENE INSTRUCTION

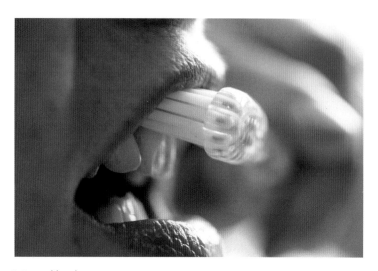

Figure 2.2 Toothbrushing

is immaterial as long as the plaque is removed. Disclosing agents can be used to determine the most successful method for a patient.

When performed thoroughly, manual brushing is just as effective as that completed with electric brushing, but the latter takes the effort out of good brushing for those patients who lack the time and skill to perform manual brushing well.

When toothbrushing is combined with the application of a fluoridated toothpaste, the teeth and gums are cleaned free of plaque and the teeth are protected from dental caries by the action of fluoride on the enamel.

Details of procedure

The aim of good toothbrushing is to remove plaque from the gingival margins, and to protect the tooth surface with a layer of fluoride.

Many toothpastes are available to patients (fluoridated, tartar controlling, desensitising, whitening, etc.), and the oral health team will advise the most suitable in each case.

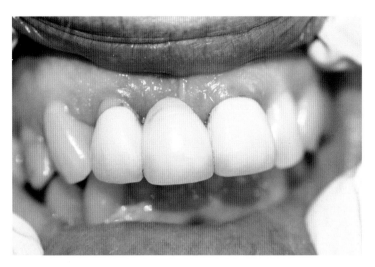

Figure 2.3 Recession over bridge abutment from heavy toothbrushing

Similarly, many toothbrush designs are available – both manual and electric – but, as a general rule, the head should be small to allow easy manoeuvrability, and the bristles should be multitufted and made of medium nylon. Even so, some patients brush with such force that they actually saw into the necks of their teeth and produce abrasion cavities or cause gingival recession (see **Figure 2.3**).

Technique

- Identify those patients with regular residual plaque after toothbrushing

- Wet the patient's own brush, apply a small amount of toothpaste and allow the patient to brush his or her teeth in the usual way and in the usual time

- Disclose the plaque to identify the areas of continued accumulation

- Develop a more thorough technique with the patient to remove all the plaque

- This may involve a change of brush from manual to electric, or vice versa, as well as a change of brushing technique by the patient

- Once an effective technique has been identified, a methodical approach should be developed so that a routine brushing technique is carried out every day

- This tends to be more effective if the more difficult areas are tackled first, such as the lingual surfaces of the lower teeth

- The patient then brushes all the teeth in a systematic manner, starting in the same place and ending in the same place each time

- Advice can then be given on the frequency of brushing – usually twice daily as a minimum, but some patients may continue with a high sugar diet and need to brush after each meal

- Full dietary advice should also be discussed and ideally adjusted where necessary

- Toothbrushes should be replaced once the bristles start to splay, as they will not remove plaque effectively when worn down

INTERDENTAL CLEANING

Background information of procedure

The surfaces of the teeth that remain untouched by toothbrushing are the contact points, or interdental areas. Plaque accumulates here just as easily as on the flat surfaces of the teeth, and even more so when restorations extend into the interdental areas as, microscopically, they provide more potential for stagnation areas to occur.

Although toothbrushes are too large to clean interdentally, other oral health products have been designed to do so:

- Tape or floss

- Manual interdental brushes (see **Figure 2.4**)

- Dental woodsticks

- Some electric toothbrush heads

- Some mouthwashes

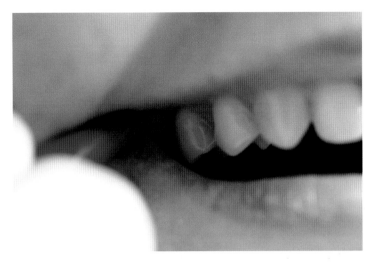

Figure 2.4 Interdental brushing

The first four are used to physically clean plaque from the interdental areas, whereas some mouthwashes can be vigorously rinsed and swished through the interdental areas by the patient to dislodge larger particles of debris.

A certain amount of manual dexterity is required by the patient to use dental tape or floss effectively, and a lack of this is often the cause of patients abandoning the technique. Some products have been developed to help, whereby a fork design holds a small piece of tape or floss firmly whilst it is used with one hand to enter and clean the interdental areas. This removes the need by the patient to wrap the tape around the fingers and to hold it firmly whilst trying to access the interdental areas.

Details of procedure

Flossing is the technique used by the majority of patients who routinely clean interdentally, despite being the most difficult to achieve.

Some tapes and flosses are waxed to assist easier entry into tight interdental areas, and others are impregnated with fluoride so that the interdental surfaces of the teeth are protected once accessed.

Technique

- Ideally, the patient should carry out flossing with the aid of a mirror in a well-lit room

- A piece of tape or floss (approximately 20 cm) is removed from the holder and wrapped around both index fingers, leaving a central portion between the hands

- This is held over both thumb pads and guided into each interdental area, one at a time

- Once in the area, the thumbs are used to adapt the tape to the surface of one tooth and then the other forming the contact point

- Whilst in contact with the tooth surface, the tape is drawn from side to side to wipe any plaque from each surface

- As the tape is dirtied, it is loaded off one finger and onto the other, so that a clean portion is available for the next interdental area

- Tape is more gentle than floss on the gingivae if the patient is heavy handed or if force is required to access tight interdental areas, but some patients may find tape too thick to use effectively

SECTION 3
SCALING AND POLISHING

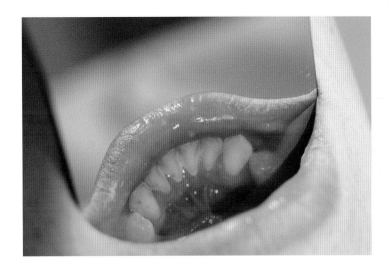

REASON FOR PROCEDURE

Everyone's mouth contains a variety of bacteria, some of which react with saliva and the food that is eaten to produce a sticky film, called plaque. Plaque forms wherever food debris becomes lodged in the mouth, usually along the gum margin and in areas that are difficult to clean, called stagnation areas.

Plaque lying along the gum margin will irritate the soft tissue and eventually cause inflammation of the gum, or gingivitis. Regular toothbrushing and interdental cleaning by the patient will remove the plaque and prevent this from happening.

However, if the plaque is not removed, it gradually hardens by absorbing minerals from the patient's saliva and becomes calculus (tartar). Calculus cannot be removed by toothbrushing alone, and the dentist or hygienist will need to remove it by scaling the teeth.

If the calculus is left untouched, it gradually forms further and further down the side of the tooth root as the gum tissue is destroyed, and eventually the supporting structures of the tooth (the jaw bone and periodontal ligaments) are also destroyed and the tooth becomes loose in its socket. This is called periodontal disease, or periodontitis (see **Figure 3.1**).

SCALING AND POLISHING

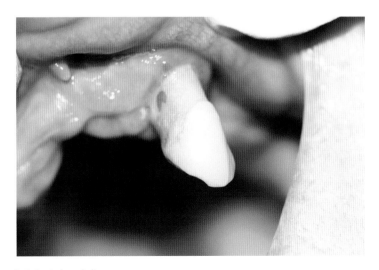

Figure 3.1 Periodontal disease

The more advanced the damage to the periodontal tissues, the more difficult it is for the dentist to treat, and the more likely that long-term problems, including tooth loss, will occur.

The procedures to be discussed are:

- Scaling

- Polishing

SCALING

Background information of procedure

The dentist or hygienist can scale a patient's teeth using hand instruments or electric scalers, or a combination of both. The aim of the procedure is to remove all the calculus from around each tooth, so that the supporting structures are no longer irritated and inflamed, and repair themselves (see **Figures 3.2 & 3.3**).

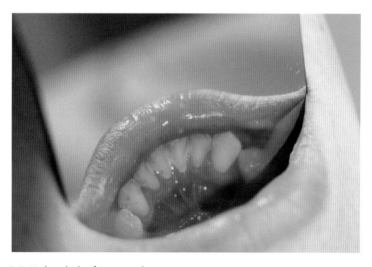

Figure 3.2 Early calculus formation, lower incisors

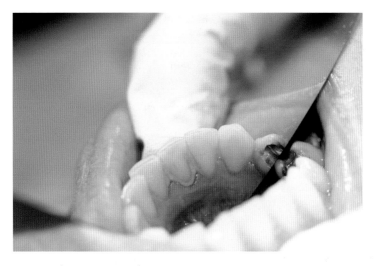

Figure 3.3 Lingual tartar at gingival margins

If the calculus has extended down the side of the root and under the gum, its removal is more difficult to achieve. Electric scalers vibrate ultrasonically and have a spray of water at their tip to help remove the calculus from both the tooth root and under the gum.

Some patients find the vibration and cold water uncomfortable, and may choose to have a scaling carried out under local anaesthetic.

Details of procedure

The presence of calculus will have been noticed by the dentist during routine examination of the patient's mouth. The amount present and whether local anaesthesia is required will help to determine whether a second appointment will be needed, or whether the scaling can be completed during the examination appointment.

Technique

- The dentist, nurse and patient wear personal protective equipment

- Local anaesthetic is given if required

- Hand and/or electric scalers are made ready

- If an electric scaler is employed, the dental nurse uses high-speed suction to remove water and debris from the patient's mouth as the scaling is carried out

- The dentist or hygienist systematically scales each tooth and root that has calculus present, using vision and tactile sensation to determine when it has been fully removed

- The scaler is worked from the bottom edge of the calculus upwards in a scraping motion, so that it is dislodged *en masse*

- The instrument is then reapplied to remove any remaining specks of calculus until a smooth tooth root surface is achieved

- The process will cause a certain amount of bleeding of the gums as they are in an inflamed state, but scaling does not cut into the gums themselves (see **Figure 3.4**)

- The gums will return to their healthy pink appearance within days of the calculus being removed

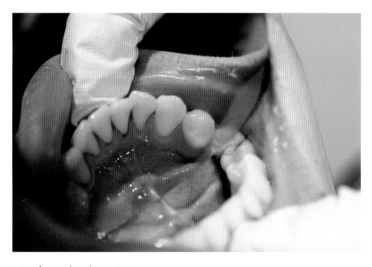

Figure 3.4 After scaling lower incisors

POLISHING

Background information of procedure

Whether or not calculus is present, everyone's teeth can stain from time to time by exposure to normal dietary substances, such as tea, coffee, red wine and highly coloured foods. Smokers can also develop unsightly dark staining from cigarette tar products.

The process of professional polishing of the anterior teeth using special abrasive pastes can easily remove all but the most tenacious of these surface stains, giving the teeth a cleaner and brighter appearance.

Obviously, continued exposure to the staining agents will cause the discolouration to develop again with time, but it can usually be kept more under control if the patient has a good and regular oral hygiene routine.

Polishing causes no surface damage to the teeth (see **Figure 3.5**).

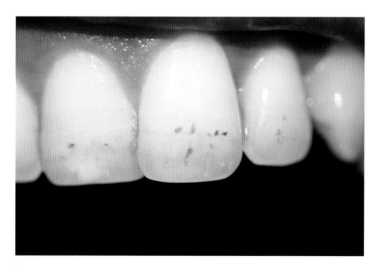

Figure 3.5 Tea stains

SCALING AND POLISHING

Details of procedure

Polishing is usually carried out at the end of a course of treatment, and especially once scaling has been completed. The use of bristle brushes or rubber cups in the dental handpiece to apply the abrasive polishing paste gives a greater cleaning effect than if it is applied, for example, using a toothbrush.

The pastes are often flavoured for the benefit of the patient, and feel quite gritty in the mouth.

Technique

- If not already in place, the dentist, nurse and patient wear personal protective equipment

- Either a bristle brush or rubber cup is locked into the dental handpiece, and is then dabbed into the polishing paste so that a small amount is picked up

- With the lips held out of the way, the rotating brush is moved across the front surface of each anterior tooth until the stains are removed

- The patient will feel a not unpleasant tickling sensation in each tooth

- The brush is worked over the whole tooth surface, and especially into the contact points of the teeth where stains usually accumulate

- Fresh paste is picked up on the brush for each tooth

- Once the procedure has been completed, the patient can rinse the gritty paste out of the mouth

SECTION 4
DIAGNOSTIC TECHNIQUES

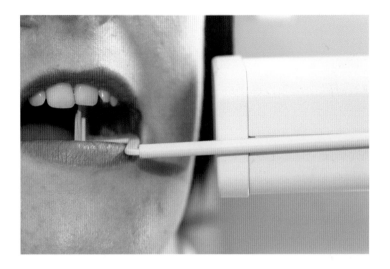

REASON FOR PROCEDURE

When a patient attends a dental appointment for a dental examination, the dentist must check his or her oral health and determine the presence of caries, periodontal disease or oral soft tissue problems. Although the visual skills of the dentist are of paramount importance in identifying problems of the oral tissues, it is often necessary for diagnostic techniques to be implemented so that a definitive diagnosis can be made.

The three techniques to be discussed are:

• Use of dental hand instruments

• Dental radiographs

• Study models

USE OF DENTAL HAND INSTRUMENTS

Background information of procedure

A variety of dental hand instruments, called probes, have been designed to aid the dentist in detecting the presence of both caries and periodontal disease.

Those used to detect caries have sharp points that can be run over the tooth surface to find any softened areas of the enamel, which indicates that demineralisation has occurred and the area has undergone carious attack.

Those used to detect periodontal disease are blunt ended and have graded depth markings on them, so that the gums are not pierced during use and any gum pockets discovered can be depth recorded.

Details of procedure – dental caries

Frank carious cavities in teeth are easily visible to the dentist when they occur on uncovered and easily accessible surfaces of the teeth, but areas that are more difficult to examine require the use of dental probes. All have been designed so that their pointed ends are bent at various angles, enabling all surfaces of each tooth to be easily probed by the dentist.

Technique

- The patient is placed in the dental chair at a suitable angle for the dentist, with the dental inspection light providing good illumination when the mouth is open

- Visual examination is carried out first, so that any suspicious tooth surfaces are detected

- Each suspect area is then revisited and the probe end is run over the tooth surface

- A hard, scratchy surface indicates sound enamel

- A soft, non-scratchy surface indicates the presence of dental caries

- The dentist will be able to determine the presence of either by tactile sensation through the probe to the hand

Details of procedure – periodontal disease

Periodontal disease is often more difficult to detect by vision alone, as the gums of some patients will appear to be quite healthy and will exhibit no bleeding on touch. The presence of periodontal pockets alongside the tooth roots indicates that some destruction of the supporting tissues of the tooth has occurred – and the deeper the pocket, the more severe the destruction.

The pockets are not visible to the naked eye, but can be easily detected using a periodontal probe (see **Figure 4.1**).

Technique

- The patient is placed in the dental chair at a suitable angle for the dentist, with the dental inspection light providing good illumination when the mouth is open

- Visual examination is carried out first, including the identification of any tooth mobility

- Each suspect tooth–gum junction is then inspected for periodontal pocketing by 'walking' the blunt-ended probe around the gingival crevice

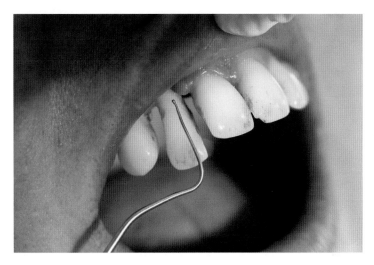

Figure 4.1 Periodontal probe out of pocket

- A healthy gingival crevice will be no deeper than 2 mm and will not bleed when probed

- Where a periodontal problem exists, the probe will sink easily below the tooth–gum junction and the area will bleed on probing (see **Figure 4.2**)

- The probe may sink for several millimetres, and greater depths indicate more severe periodontal disease

- Sometimes the probe may also detect specks of subgingival calculus on the tooth root

DENTAL RADIOGRAPHS

Background information of procedure

Radiographs provide the dentist with a method of seeing within the dental tissues themselves, without having to drill or cut into these tissues beforehand.

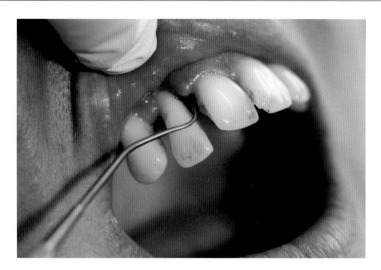

Figure 4.2 Periodontal pocket

They are an invaluable diagnostic technique for determining the presence or absence of dental disease, as well as such widely varying features as unerupted teeth, jaw or tooth fractures, extra teeth, foreign bodies and so on.

A wide variety of images can be produced depending on the type of radiographic view required, ranging from a single tooth to the whole oral cavity. When a single tooth or just a few teeth are to be viewed, an intra-oral radiograph is taken that can then either be chemically processed to produce an image or transmitted with specialist digital equipment to a computer screen for immediate viewing.

Those to be discussed are:

• Bitewings (see **Figure 4.3**)

• Periapicals (see **Figure 4.4**)

When a more extensive area is to be radiographed, an extra-oral orthopantomograph (OPT) view is taken, using a cassette containing intensifying screens to reduce the X-ray exposure of the patient (see **Figure 4.5**).

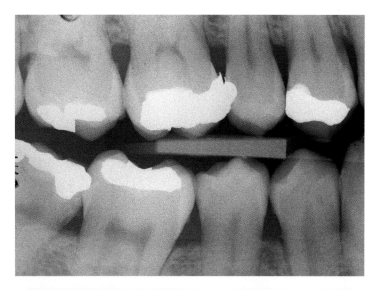

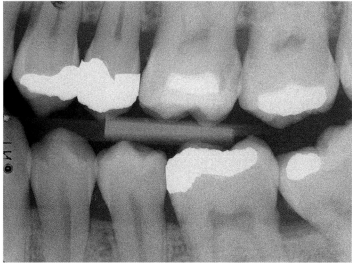

Figure 4.3 Bitewing radiographs

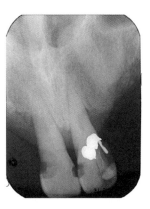

Figure 4.4 Periapical radiograph

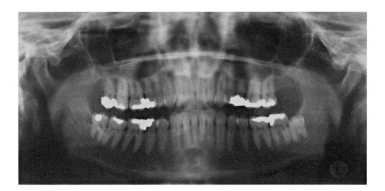

Figure 4.5 Orthopantomograph (OPT) showing full dental arches

Details of procedure

When an intra-oral view is being taken, it is important that there is no distortion of the film or the image produced, as can happen if the film is bent in the mouth or if the angulation of the X-ray machine cone is incorrect. Therefore, the film is placed into one of a variety of holders before being positioned in the patient's mouth, so that the film is held parallel to the tooth being exposed and to prevent distortion, as well as allowing the cone angulation to be set correctly.

If a digital radiograph is to be produced, the sensor unit is treated in the same manner.

Technique

- The patient is seated comfortably in the dental chair, usually in an upright position or nearly so

- All removable prostheses are taken out of the mouth, as they will superimpose their image over the teeth and make diagnosis difficult

- The X-ray machine exposure and time settings are chosen by the operator, depending on which tooth and view are being taken

- A holder is chosen depending on whether a bitewing, anterior or posterior periapical view is required (see **Figure 4.6**)

- An intra-oral film is correctly inserted into the holder so that the front of the film faces the X-ray cone

- The holder and film are then gently but accurately positioned in the patient's mouth, so that the tooth to be viewed lies between the film holder and the X-ray cone, and parallel with both (see **Figures 4.7 & 4.8**)

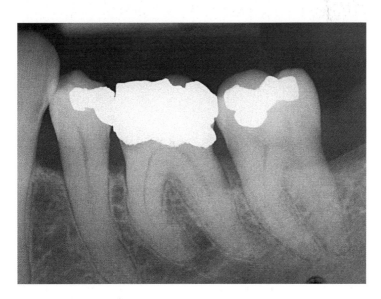

Figure 4.6 Posterior periapical view

DIAGNOSTIC TECHNIQUES

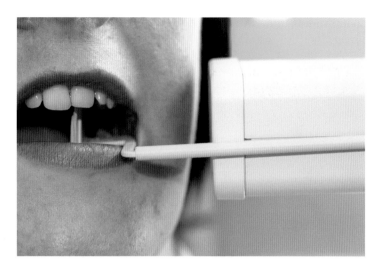

Figure 4.7 Bitewing position

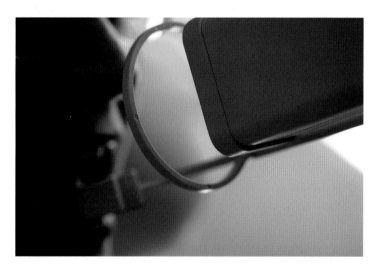

Figure 4.8 Anterior periapical position

- The final position of the X-ray cone is checked before all personnel, except the patient, move at least 1.5 m away from the exposure area

- The patient is told to remain completely still during the exposure, which is identified by a ringing or buzzing sound

- The operator presses the X-ray machine button to expose the film, releasing it only when the audio alarm ends

- A digital X-ray view will be produced immediately on the computer screen

- Ordinary film is removed from the patient's mouth and holder, and taken to be chemically processed either manually or in an automatic processor

- The processed radiograph can be viewed on a viewer within 5 min, and a diagnosis made

When an OPT is to be taken, the patient must be correctly positioned within the headset of the X-ray machine, so that the film produced is in focus throughout and no positional distortions are produced. The exposure time is usually in the region of 15 s, but a reduced X-ray dose to the patient is achieved by the use of intensifying screens within the cassette.

The film is chemically processed to produce the image, either manually or automatically. These views are often taken for orthodontic diagnosis of missing or unerupted teeth, as well as to identify jaw fractures and pathology.

STUDY MODELS

Background information of procedure

When a patient has a complicated occlusion, it is easier for the dentist to visualise this by copying the dental arches and the way in which they bite together by producing a set of study models. These can then be viewed from all angles by the dentist, without the hindrance of the patient's lips, cheeks and tongue.

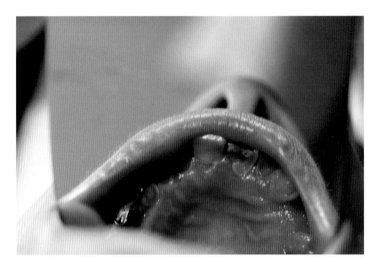

Figure 4.9 Tooth wear in bruxism

Often, unexpected details are discovered that were not evident just by viewing the patient in the dental chair, such as abnormal wear patterns on the teeth.

Diagnostic study models are invaluable aids to the dentist for the following situations:

• Orthodontics

• Multiple crown restorations

• Bridges

• Implants

• Bruxism (tooth grinding) (see **Figure 4.9**)

• Denture design

Details of procedure

When producing diagnostic study models, an impression must be taken of each arch of the patient's dentition that is accurate without being prohibitively expensive. The impression material of choice is alginate, which is sufficiently elastomeric to be accurate as well as being relatively inexpensive. Correctly sized stock trays are adequate to hold the impression material, and a wax wafer bite allows the accurate positioning of the two models produced.

In more complicated cases, the models are often mounted on an articulator so that jaw movements can be reproduced and a more in-depth occlusal analysis can be carried out.

Technique

- The patient is seated upright in a dental chair

- A protective bib is placed

- All removable prostheses are taken out of the mouth, unless their presence is required for the occlusal analysis

- A wax wafer bite is taken, if necessary, using warmed pink wax

- Upper and lower stock trays are sized to the patient's dental arches, so that each arch is fully covered by the tray without being uncomfortable or choking the patient

- A stiff, bubble-free mix of alginate is prepared, loaded into one of the trays and inserted into the patient's mouth to fully cover one of the dental arches

- The patient is advised to breathe through the nose, not to swallow and to keep the lips and cheeks in a relaxed state

- Once set, the impression is carefully removed from the mouth in the tray and disinfected as necessary

- The process is repeated for the opposing arch

- Study models are cast from the impressions in dental stone, ideally within 24 h of the impressions being taken

DIAGNOSTIC TECHNIQUES

SECTION 5

TOOTH RESTORATION WITH FILLINGS

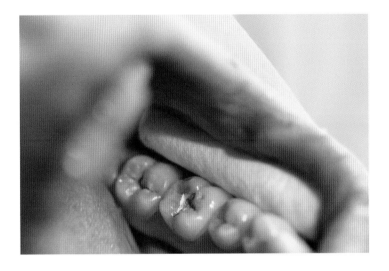

REASON FOR PROCEDURE

When a tooth is attacked by caries, a process of demineralisation occurs in the hard tissues of the tooth, starting in the enamel outer layer. This opens up the inner dentine layer to infection by the bacteria involved in caries and, as this layer contains nerve endings, the patient will feel hot and cold sensitivity and eventually pain. Once painful, there will be a loss of function as the patient avoids chewing with the affected tooth.

The caries attack will progress further into the tooth until it reaches the pulp chamber, eventually causing an abscess and the death of the tooth, unless the tooth is dentally treated by filling (see **Figure 5.1a, b**).

A tooth may also require a filling if it fractures, whether or not caries is involved, as a fractured tooth may also become sensitive to hot and cold, or cause soft tissue trauma to areas within the oral cavity (see **Figure 5.2**).

The purpose of the filling procedure is ultimately to restore the tooth to its normal function, and this will involve the elimination of any caries first, as well as the elimination of any discomfort or pain experienced by the patient.

The procedures to be discussed are:

- Amalgam fillings

- Composite fillings

- Glass ionomer fillings

AMALGAM FILLINGS

Background information of procedure

Amalgam is a metallic material used for fillings, produced by the mixing of an alloy powder (containing mainly silver) with a small amount of liquid mercury. This produces a plastic material that can be inserted fully into the tooth cavity and then carved to the shape of the tooth surface. Once set, it forms a solid plug in the cavity that is hard enough to chew on, as well as

TOOTH RESTORATION WITH FILLINGS

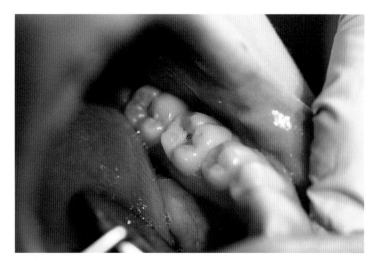

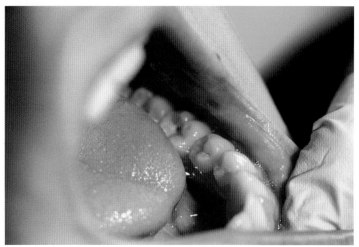

Figure 5.1 (a, b) Caries in lower first molar

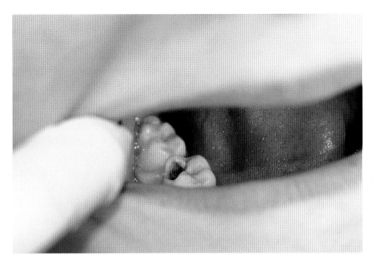

Figure 5.2 Fractured carious tooth

sealing the tooth's sensitive inner layers from further exposure to hot and cold stimulants.

As the material is metallic in appearance, it tends not to be used for anterior fillings, as far more acceptable aesthetics are produced here using tooth-coloured filling materials.

Details of procedure

The procedure is normally carried out under local anaesthetic, so that the patient feels neither pain nor thermal stimulation in the tooth. The effects of the local anaesthetic will wear off after several hours, by which time the dental treatment will have been completed painlessly.

During the procedure, a dental nurse provides good moisture control in the oral cavity using high-speed suction equipment, so that the dentist has a clear field of vision at all times. The suction equipment is used to remove saliva, debris from the tooth and water from the dental handpiece that cools the drill whilst in use.

Technique

- The dentist, nurse and patient wear personal protective equipment for safety reasons; this usually consists of goggles and mask for the dental team, and a protective bib and safety glasses for the patient

- Local anaesthetic is administered and allowed to take full effect

- All caries is removed from the tooth cavity using a combination of high- and low-speed dental handpieces with drills, and cutting hand instruments

- This produces a firm tooth cavity surface into which the filling can be placed, which is then undercut to prevent loss of the completed filling

- Depending on the depth of the finished cavity, a protective lining may be placed over the base so that the pulp beneath is not exposed to thermal irritation through the metallic filling

- If more than one tooth surface has been destroyed by caries, a metal matrix band is placed around the tooth and tightened to allow the amalgam to be pushed into the cavity from one surface without squeezing out of the other

- The mixed amalgam is inserted into the cavity in increments by the dental team, starting at its deepest point and gradually filling the cavity to the surface of the tooth

- After each increment, the dentist uses hand instruments to push the plastic amalgam material into all the cavity depths so that no voids remain – these would weaken the filling and allow future fracture

- The dental nurse uses high-speed suction to remove all excess amalgam from the area, as the dentist carves and shapes the surface of the filling

- Once completed, the shape of the filling should allow the patient to bite together without prematurely contacting it, but so that the tooth can still be used for chewing (see **Figure 5.3**)

- The patient is advised not to attempt chewing until the local anaesthetic has worn off to avoid the risk of biting himself or herself

- By this time, the amalgam will be hardened and fully set

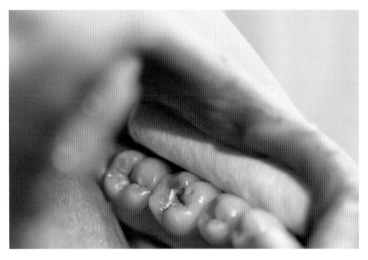

Figure 5.3 Amalgam filling

COMPOSITE FILLINGS

Background information of procedure

Composite is a tooth-coloured filling material that is available in many shades to match a very wide range of tooth colours. It can be polished, once set, to produce a shiny surface that matches tooth enamel superbly, and is therefore an excellent material to be used for anterior fillings. Some modern types of composite are also strong and sufficiently wear resistant to be used as a posterior filling material instead of amalgam.

Unlike amalgam, composite is not freshly mixed and does not set with time; rather, it is used in its ready-mixed plastic state to fill a cavity, and then set (or cured) by exposure to a blue curing lamp. This gives the dentist more time to fully adapt the plastic material to the tooth as required, before using the curing lamp to harden it in a controlled manner.

Although composite is far superior to amalgam aesthetically, it can take longer to use and the procedure is technique sensitive.

Details of procedure

Again, local anaesthesia is usually administered before dental treatment begins, and a dental nurse provides moisture control throughout the procedure as composite is particularly sensitive to moisture contamination.

Indeed, some dentists choose to isolate the tooth completely from the rest of the oral cavity whilst placing composite fillings by using a rubber dam. This allows the tooth to be restored to project through the rubber dam sheet whilst keeping all other oral structures away from it, thus preventing saliva contamination of the tooth whilst the filling is placed.

Technique

- The dentist, nurse and patient wear personal protective equipment, and, ideally, the patient's safety glasses should be orange tinted to counteract the blue curing lamp

- Local anaesthetic is administered and allowed to take full effect

- A rubber dam is placed if required

- All caries is removed from the tooth cavity as before, but then the preparation is minimal as the composite material bonds to enamel and no undercuts are required to hold the filling in place

- A lining may be placed in deeper cavities to prevent chemical irritation of the pulp by the filling material

- The required shade is chosen using a shade guide in natural light (this may be taken beforehand if a rubber dam is placed)

- The exposed enamel edges of the cavity are covered in acid etch to chemically roughen their surfaces

- The etch is washed off, the edges are dried and unfilled resin is wiped over them and cured with a blue lamp for a short time

- The resin will form a bond between the enamel and the filling material, locking the latter into place

- A transparent matrix strip is used to avoid overspill as the composite is placed into the cavity, in 2 mm increments, that are individually cured to ensure full setting of the overall filling

- The matrix is transparent to allow the curing light beam to pass through it

- Coloured articulating paper is used to identify any premature contacts on any biting surfaces of the filling, and these are removed to allow the patient to achieve his or her correct bite

- Polishing strips, discs and burrs are used to produce the final shiny surface of the completed filling

- Although the filling is fully set once cured, the patient is advised not to attempt chewing until the local anaesthetic has worn off

GLASS IONOMER FILLINGS

Background information of procedure

Glass ionomer is another tooth-coloured filling material available for tooth restoration, although the shade range is more limited than for composite. It is also less translucent and cannot be polished to give a shiny surface, and so the final aesthetics produced are inferior to composite.

The advantage of glass ionomer over other filling materials is that it is adhesive to all tooth surfaces – enamel, dentine and cementum – and is therefore invaluable in filling cavities where minimal if any tooth preparation is possible. This is a particular advantage when filling abrasion cavities produced at the necks of the teeth, often by overzealous toothbrushing by the patient.

It is also useful in filling the deciduous teeth of young patients who often will not tolerate the administration of local anaesthetic. It is of special value here as it releases fluoride into the cavity and helps to slow or stop the progression of caries.

It is usually provided as a powder of glass-like material which is mixed by hand with an acidic liquid, or as a capsule containing both agents that are mixed mechanically; some forms set chemically with time, whereas others set after exposure to a blue curing lamp. Attempts to adjust the surface of the filling once set produce a chalky appearance, and so accurate placement of a light-cured type requiring no adjustment will produce the best aesthetic result.

Details of procedure

As little or no tooth preparation is required with this material unless caries is present, local anaesthesia may not always be needed. However, good moisture control is imperative to allow the filling to set properly, and so a rubber dam may well be placed in adult patients.

Technique

- The dentist, nurse and patient wear personal protective equipment

- Local anaesthetic is administered if caries removal is necessary

- A rubber dam is placed if required

- Any caries is fully removed if present; otherwise, no tooth preparation is required

- The cavity is conditioned by wiping it fully with polyacrylic liquid to remove dirt and any preparation debris and to allow chemical bonding of the filling to the tooth

- The conditioner is washed off and the cavity is dried

- Deeper cavities are lined to prevent chemical irritation of the pulp

- The mixed filling material is applied and fully adapted to the cavity so that no adjustment is required once set

- Light-cured types of glass ionomer are cured as necessary, whereas chemically cured types are kept dry whilst setting occurs with time

- The set surface is coated with a waterproof varnish to prevent the filling drying out once set

AFTERCARE OF FILLINGS

No matter how well placed, microscopically, the edges of a filling provide a new surface area for plaque and oral bacteria to adhere to, giving the potential for further carious attack if not removed regularly (see **Figures 5.4a, b & 5.5**).

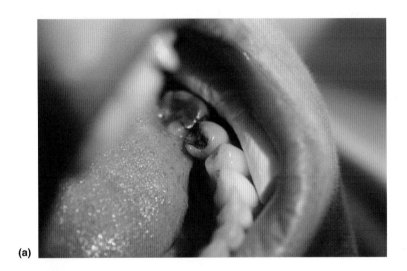

(a)

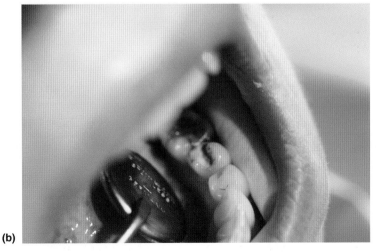

(b)

Figure 5.4 (a) Leaking amalgam filling. (b) New filling

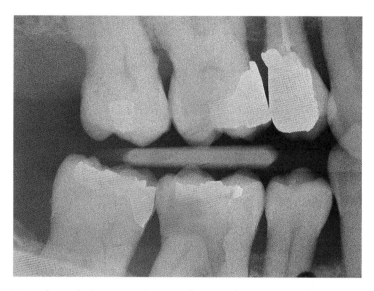

Figure 5.5 Radiograph showing amalgam overhang as plaque retention factor

Consistently high standards of oral hygiene must be maintained by the patient to prevent this happening, and especially interdentally if the filling extends between the teeth. This will involve the use of a good toothbrushing technique with a good quality fluoridated toothpaste, as well as floss, tape or interdental brushes. Ideally, a plaque-suppressing mouthwash should also be used routinely.

The standard of oral hygiene achieved should be monitored and reinforced as necessary at regular dental examinations. Where techniques are poor and calculus has developed, this should be fully removed by scaling and polishing the teeth.

Similarly, the patient should be advised to alter his or her diet when caries has been experienced previously. The intake of foods and drinks high in refined sugars or acids should be reduced as far as possible, and confined to mealtimes to allow the natural buffering action of saliva to minimise any carious attack.

Failure to comply with these oral health instructions is likely to result in further caries and the need for further fillings in the future.

TOOTH RESTORATION WITH CROWNS, BRIDGES OR VENEERS

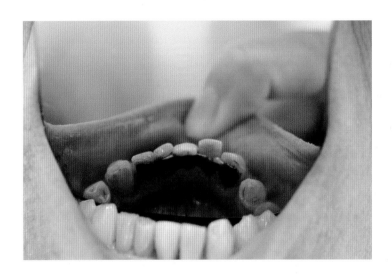

REASON FOR PROCEDURE

Each time a tooth is restored with a filling some of the tooth tissue is removed. Eventually, this will compromise the strength of the remaining tooth and it may begin to fracture under normal occlusal forces. This occurs especially when teeth have been root treated, and so it is usual for heavily filled and root-filled teeth to be crowned before fracture occurs.

In other cases, a tooth may be poorly shaped and require elective crowning to be more aesthetically pleasing. Similarly, a tooth may be too poorly shaped to assist in the retention of, for example, a denture, but this can be made possible by elective crowning.

CROWNS

Background information of procedure

Posterior crowns are usually constructed from non-precious or precious metals, such as gold (see **Figure 6.1**). These provide maximum strength to withstand occlusal forces and have no risk of fracture. Anterior crowns are made of either tooth-coloured ceramic or porcelain throughout, or have

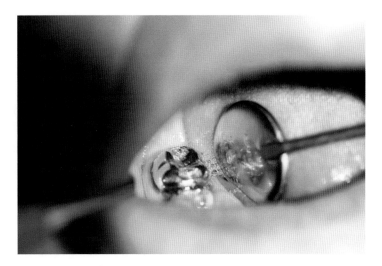

Figure 6.1 Full gold crown

TOOTH RESTORATION WITH
CROWNS, BRIDGES OR VENEERS

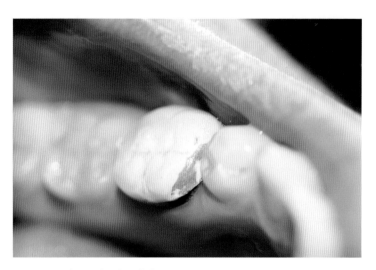

Figure 6.2 Fractured porcelain bonded crown

porcelain bonded to a substructure of metal, and these give an aesthetically pleasing result when shaded and matched accurately to the adjacent teeth. Although modern techniques of crown construction are superb, it is possible for ceramic crowns to fracture or break away from their metallic substructure, so that repairs or even replacements are required. This can occur in patients with especially heavy bites or in those who grind their teeth (see **Figure 6.2**).

Details of procedure

Unless the tooth to be crowned has been root treated and is therefore non-vital, crown preparation is usually carried out under local anaesthetic so that the patient feels neither pain nor thermal stimulation in the tooth throughout the procedure.

As the crown must be individually constructed by a technician, the prepared tooth will require thermal protection in the meantime by being covered with a temporary crown material, such as acrylic.

During the preparation procedure, a dental nurse maintains good moisture control in the oral cavity using high-speed suction equipment. This provides a clear field of vision for the dentist, as well as making the patient more comfortable by removing water, saliva and tooth debris from the mouth.

Technique

- The dentist, nurse and patient wear personal protective equipment

- Local anaesthetic is administered and allowed to take full effect

- The shade and shape of crown are chosen by the dentist and patient

- A rubber dam is placed if required

- All sides and occlusal surfaces of the tooth are reduced by a uniform amount using a burr in the high-speed handpiece, so that space is created for the crown to be constructed and fitted without altering the patient's occlusion

- The side reduction is completed to produce a near-parallel tooth core in order to give maximum retention of the crown on cementation

- Once tooth preparation is complete, impressions are taken of both arches and the patient's normal biting position is recorded

- The impression of the opposing arch can be taken in alginate, but that of the working arch must be in a very accurate, non-tearing, elastomeric material, such as a silicone or polyether

- When satisfactory impressions have been produced, the tooth core is coated with a temporary acrylic material to prevent sensitivity and to restore some degree of aesthetics whilst the permanent crown is constructed

- Once the crown has been constructed, the patient reattends for its cementation

- Again, local anaesthetic is administered and a rubber dam is placed if required

- On removal of the temporary material, the crown is placed onto the tooth core and checked for accuracy of fit, shade and occlusion

- If satisfactory, the crown is cemented permanently onto the tooth core using one of a variety of luting cements, taking great care to ensure all excess cement is removed (see **Figure 6.3**)

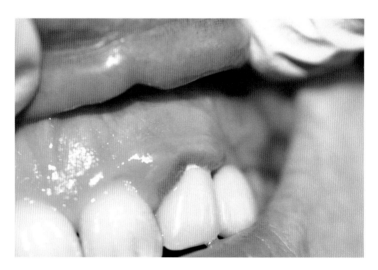

Figure 6.3 Localised gingivitis owing to incomplete cement removal at crown fit

AFTERCARE OF CROWNS

As with fillings, microscopically, all fixed prosthetic restorations provide a surface area for the attachment of plaque and oral bacteria. As crown margins are deliberately placed at the gingival margin to give superior aesthetics, any plaque accumulation can potentially cause either caries of the underlying tooth core or periodontal disease down the root of the tooth (see **Figure 6.4**).

A consistently high standard of oral hygiene around crown margins is therefore imperative. This will involve good toothbrushing using a good quality fluoride toothpaste, and successful interdental cleaning using floss or tape. As many crowns are placed specifically to close existing interdental spaces, it is unlikely that the use of interdental brushes will be possible.

Regular use of a plaque-suppressing mouthwash should also be encouraged, and the oral hygiene standard achieved by the patient can be monitored and reinforced at regular dental examinations. Any calculus found to be present should be fully removed by scaling and polishing the teeth.

As always, a diet high in sugars and acids should be reduced to an absolute minimum, and confined to mealtimes only.

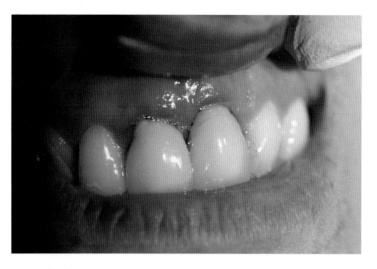

Figure 6.4 Localised gingivitis at crown margin

BRIDGES

Background information of procedure

A bridge is a fixed restoration used to replace one or a few missing teeth in a dental arch, although, in advanced cases, multiple bridges can be fitted to provide full mouth rehabilitation.

Various designs of bridge are available, and each case must be determined on its merits.

In patients with a few missing teeth and a low biting force in the area of the bridge, a minimal amount of tooth preparation can be carried out and an acid etch retained bridge can be placed (see **Figure 6.5**). Where occlusal forces are likely to dislodge this type of restoration, a more conventional design is used in which the adjacent teeth are prepared as for crowns and the missing teeth are incorporated into the whole structure (see **Figures 6.6 & 6.7**).

Bridges are usually constructed of porcelain bonded to a metallic substructure, although some modern all-ceramic materials are also available.

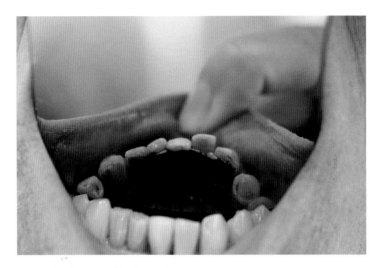

Figure 6.5 Acid-etch retained bridge

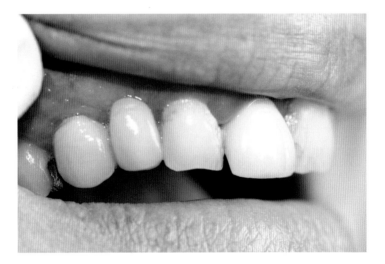

Figure 6.6 Example of two-unit cantilever bridge

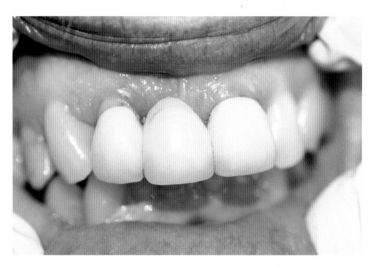

Figure 6.7 Example of three-unit fixed bridge

Details of procedure

As minimal tooth preparation is carried out for an acid etch bridge, it is often not necessary for local anaesthetic to be administered. With more conventional designs involving whole tooth preparation, it is usual for local anaesthetic to be administered for any vital teeth involved.

As always, a dental nurse provides good moisture control in the oral cavity throughout the bridge preparation procedure.

Technique

- The dentist, nurse and patient wear personal protective equipment

- Local anaesthetic is administered, if necessary, and allowed to take full effect

- The design of bridge will already have been discussed and decided upon by the dentist and patient, and the shade will be chosen now

- A rubber dam is placed if required

- If an acid etch bridge is being provided, a small area of enamel at the back of the retaining adjacent teeth is removed to provide room for the technician to construct the retaining metal wings that will hold the bridge in place

- These must be constructed so as not to interfere with the patient's normal occlusion

- When a more conventional bridge is being provided, each retaining tooth is reduced to a core, as for a crown preparation, using the same technique and design principles

- Once prepared, an impression of the working arch is taken in a highly accurate material, such as silicone or polyether, and one of the opposing arch is taken in alginate

- The bite and jaw movements can be recorded simply, or with the help of articulated study models, depending on the complexity of the case

- The prepared teeth are temporarily covered to prevent sensitivity, as with crown preparations

- In complex cases, the metallic substructure of the bridge (if used) is placed for accuracy of fit before the porcelain is bonded to it, as this avoids costly full remakes if problems occur

- Once the bridge has been fully constructed, the patient reattends for its cementation

- Local anaesthetic is administered and a rubber dam is placed if necessary

- On removal of the temporary coverings, the bridge is placed onto the retaining teeth and checked for accuracy of fit, shade and occlusion

- The replaced missing tooth (or teeth) is checked for its fit against the bony ridge of the dental arch, to ensure that the area will be easily cleaned by the patient

- Once satisfactory, an acid etch retained bridge is cemented using one of a variety of light-cured bonding materials

- A conventional bridge is cemented using one of a variety of luting cements

AFTERCARE OF BRIDGES

All of the aftercare advice for crowns is similarly applicable to bridges, but additional oral hygiene techniques need to be employed when maintaining the pontic areas of a bridge (see **Figures 6.8 & 6.9**).

The point at which the pontic rests on the gingiva is a difficult area to clean, and may accumulate plaque and oral bacteria quite easily. This will cause gingival inflammation unless the plaque is removed, either by vigorous mouthwashing or by physically cleaning the underside of the pontic using floss or tape (see **Figure 6.10**).

Where the pontic has retainers on both sides so that the bridge is a solid structure, superfloss can be threaded beneath the pontic and used to clean its underside. Superfloss has a stiff end for threading, which is attached to an expanded spongy section that then runs into normal floss. It has been designed specifically to clean bridges in this way.

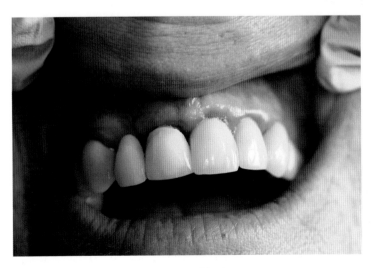

Figure 6.8 Periodontal disease developing around bridge

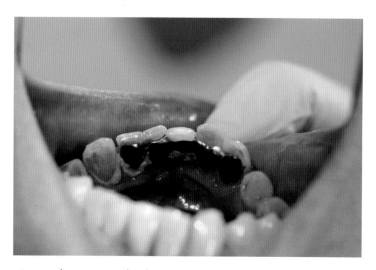

Figure 6.9 Lingual tartar accumulated around bridge

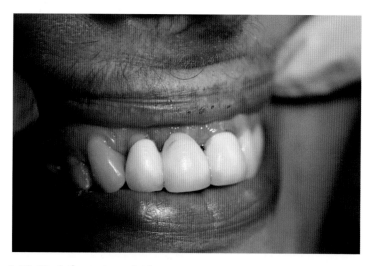

Figure 6.10 Gingival recession at bridge retainer

VENEERS

Background information of procedure

A less invasive technique than conventional crown preparation for improving the aesthetics of a tooth is to place a veneer. These are thin layers of porcelain that are acid etch cemented to the front surface of any number of anterior teeth to improve a patient's appearance by correcting dark or malaligned teeth, or both (see **Figure 6.11**).

They have no other functional purpose other than cosmetic, and their fragility and ease of fracture or loss dictate their case suitability. Patients with aberrant occlusal habits or heavy bites are usually unsuitable for veneers.

Although usually constructed of porcelain, it is possible to place either composite or acrylic veneers on a temporary basis.

Details of procedure

As minimal tooth preparation is carried out for a veneer, it is often not necessary for local anaesthetic to be administered. Indeed, it is frequently root-filled, discoloured teeth that have veneers placed to improve aesthetics, as full crown

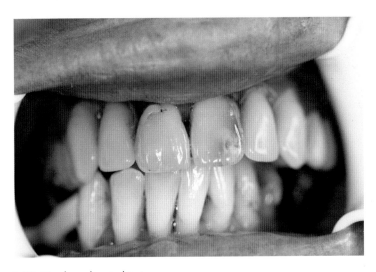

Figure 6.11 Discoloured central incisors

TOOTH RESTORATION WITH CROWNS, BRIDGES OR VENEERS

preparations on these teeth can sometimes compromise them sufficiently to cause fracture with time.

A dental nurse provides good moisture control in the oral cavity throughout the veneer preparation procedure.

Technique

- The dentist, nurse and patient wear personal protective equipment

- Local anaesthetic is administered, as necessary, and allowed to take full effect

- The shade and shape of the veneer are chosen by the dentist and patient, as is the need for any opaquing technique if a particularly dark tooth is involved

- A rubber dam is placed if required

- The labial (front) surface of each tooth to be veneered is reduced uniformly using a burr in the high-speed handpiece (see **Figure 6.12**)

- This is to provide the technician with sufficient space to construct the veneer, so that the restoration remains in line with the adjacent teeth, rather than projecting further forwards than required

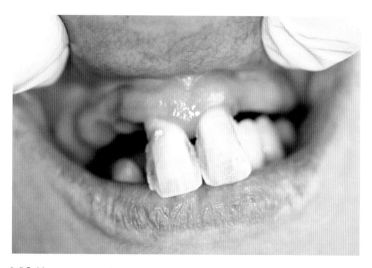

Figure 6.12 Veneer preparations

- Once the veneer preparation is complete, a highly accurate working impression is taken in a material such as silicone or polyether

- If the occlusion of the prepared tooth has been altered, an opposing alginate impression and bite record are also taken

- The prepared surface can be temporarily covered with composite to avoid sensitivity and to improve aesthetics, but this is sometimes not carried out with non-vital teeth

- Once the veneer has been constructed, the patient reattends for its cementation

- Local anaesthetic is administered and a rubber dam is placed if required

- On removal of any temporary covering, the veneer is placed onto the tooth and checked for accuracy of fit, shade and shape

- The final shade can be accurately achieved by the use of various tooth-coloured cements if necessary

- The veneer is secured to the tooth using one of a variety of light-cured bonding materials (see **Figure 6.13**)

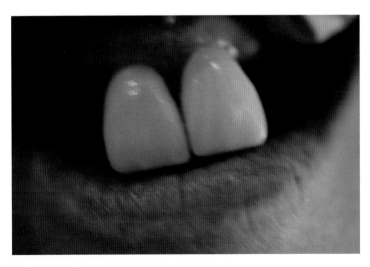

Figure 6.13 Veneer fits

TOOTH RESTORATION WITH
CROWNS, BRIDGES OR VENEERS

AFTERCARE OF VENEERS

As with other restorations, veneers can be subject to plaque and oral bacteria accumulations at their margins. Their aftercare advice is similar to that for crowns, whereby a consistently good standard of plaque removal is required to prevent caries developing at the veneer margins and periodontal problems developing at the gingival margins.

This is achieved using a thorough toothbrushing technique with fluoride toothpaste, careful interdental cleaning using floss or tape, and the regular use of a plaque-suppressing mouthwash.

Regular dental examinations should be carried out, where oral hygiene techniques can be reinforced as necessary, and any scaling and polishing can be performed to remove any accumulated calculus deposits.

Dietary advice should include a reduction in the intake of sugars and acids to a minimum, and at mealtimes only.

TOOTH RESTORATION WITH
CROWNS, BRIDGES OR VENEERS

SECTION 7
TOOTH RESTORATION WITH ENDODONTIC TECHNIQUES

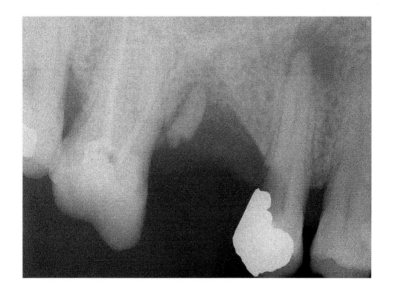

REASON FOR PROCEDURE

Any event that places the pulp tissue within the root canal of a tooth at risk of inflammation or infection may eventually lead to the death of that tooth. Once a tooth has died, it is a source of either painless chronic infection or acute and very painful infection, neither of which are amenable to the oral health of a patient.

Events that can result in the inflammation of the pulp (pulpitis) include the following:

* Deep caries lying close to, or exposing, the pulp (see **Figure 7.1**)

* Thermal injury

* Chemical irritation from restorative materials

* Trauma, which may be severe enough to cause tooth fracture in some cases

* Prolonged irritation from very deep fillings

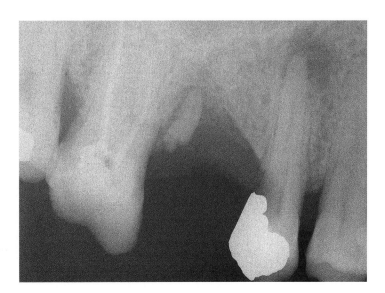

Figure 7.1 Radiograph showing deep caries and periapical area

TOOTH RESTORATION WITH
ENDODONTIC TECHNIQUES

The only methods available to the dentist to remove the symptoms, treat the tooth and save it from extraction are as follows:

- Pulp capping

- Pulpotomy

- Pulpectomy

PULP CAPPING

Background information of procedure

This is a technique carried out as a temporary measure to stabilise the tooth before proceeding to either pulpotomy or pulpectomy to save it from extraction. It is necessary when a small pulp exposure occurs unexpectedly during restorative dental treatment, or when a patient attends as an unscheduled emergency following trauma.

The aim of pulp capping is to seal the exposed pulp from the oral cavity, and the myriad of microorganisms within it, until time allows for a full endodontic procedure to be carried out to save the tooth.

Details of procedure

If pulp exposure occurs during restorative treatment, it is likely that a local anaesthetic will have been administered previously. If a recent trauma has caused the exposure, the tooth is likely to be concussed and unresponsive to stimulation.

In any event, the tooth must be kept as clean as possible to prevent the introduction of microorganisms into the pulp chamber. Once completed, pulp capping will prevent pain and infection developing before further treatment can be carried out.

Technique

- The dentist, nurse and patient wear personal protective equipment

- The tooth is isolated from saliva contamination using moisture control techniques

- Any bleeding at the exposure site is arrested using sterile cotton wool pledgets, possibly soaked in a local anaesthetic solution containing a vasoconstrictor

- Once bleeding has been arrested and the area is dry, a paste of calcium hydroxide is carefully placed over the exposure site

- The remaining cavity or fracture site is then sealed with a sedative temporary dressing material

PULPOTOMY

Background information of procedure

When trauma occurs to a permanent tooth in a child, it is often the case that the root canal is still wide open at the apex. This can be determined by radiograph.

When this is the case, the tooth often does not die as a result of trauma, as the wide apex ensures that a good blood supply to the pulp is maintained during the inflammatory process, and pulpal death is avoided. In these cases only, the potentially infected part of the pulp at the exposure site needs to be removed, and the apical blood supply will ensure that the remainder of the pulp tissue heals itself.

The partial removal of pulp tissue from the pulp chamber only, and not the root canal, is called pulpotomy.

Details of procedure

As the pulp tissue is still vital, local anaesthetic is required for the procedure. It is important to the success of the technique that any risk of contamination of the remaining pulp tissue is kept to an absolute minimum, and so the dental nurse provides good moisture control throughout.

Technique

- The dentist, nurse and patient wear personal protective equipment

- Local anaesthetic is administered and allowed to take full effect

- The tooth is isolated from saliva contamination, ideally using a rubber dam, but this may not be possible in a young patient

- The pulp chamber is opened through the fracture site using a burr in the high-speed handpiece

- The pulp tissue, within the pulp chamber only, is separated from that in the root canal using sharp, sterile hand instruments or a sterile burr in the low-speed handpiece

- Any bleeding of the amputated pulp stump is arrested using sterile cotton wool pledgets, possibly soaked in a vasoconstrictive local anaesthetic solution

- Once dry, the pulp stump is covered with a calcium hydroxide material that will encourage the formation of a protective layer of secondary dentine to grow with time, and seal off the pulp tissue in the root canal

- A stiff base material is placed over the calcium hydroxide to further protect the remaining pulp tissue from the oral environment

- The fracture site is then restored to full function and aesthetics using one of the permanent restorative filling materials

- Depending on the degree of success of the technique, it may eventually be necessary to carry out a full root-filling procedure on the tooth, but, in the meantime, the pulpotomy will have allowed the root apex to close

PULPECTOMY

Background information of procedure

When a permanent tooth undergoes an event causing inflammation in an adult patient, the end result is usually the death of the tooth. The closed root apex of an adult tooth prevents an adequate blood flow from helping to fight the inflammation and remove the excess fluids that build up during the inflammatory process. The ensuing swelling compresses the pulpal tissues and tooth death occurs. An infection will develop at the root apex that will be visible on a periapical radiograph as a circular black area (see **Figure 7.1**).

The patient will experience varying degrees of pain and swelling throughout the tooth death process, and only a successful pulpectomy procedure will avoid the extraction of the affected tooth.

The aim of pulpectomy, or root canal treatment, is to remove all of the pulpal tissue from the tooth and replace it with a sterile root-filling material. This material must fully seal the root canal and prevent any contamination from causing further infection at the root apex.

Details of procedure

Although a dead tooth should be unable to feel pain, many patients will be more psychologically comfortable and relaxed during the procedure if a local anaesthetic is administered. The success of the pulpectomy technique depends very much on the maintenance of a sterile field to prevent contamination of the root canal system with saliva and oral microorganisms, and good moisture control is of paramount importance.

Often the full root canal treatment is carried out in one appointment, but, if heavy infection is present or other difficulties occur, it may be completed in further visits.

Technique

- The dentist, nurse and patient wear personal protective equipment

- Local anaesthetic is administered, as required, and allowed to take full effect

- The tooth is isolated from the oral cavity, ideally by a rubber dam

- Access is gained to the pulp chamber and root canal system using a burr in the high-speed handpiece

- All pulpal tissue is removed (extirpated) from the tooth using specialised endodontic barbed broach instruments

- The root canal system is enlarged laterally and to the root apex using endodontic reamers, either by hand or with a low-speed handpiece

- The walls of the root canal are smoothed using endodontic files to remove any infected tissue and surface irregularities that could harbour microorganisms in the future, again either by hand or using a low-speed handpiece

- The root canal is irrigated throughout the preparation procedure to remove loose debris, lubricate the area and avoid instrument fracture

- Once the root canal system has been satisfactorily cleaned to the root apex and widened sufficiently to allow root filling, the decision is made as to whether to continue in a one-stage technique or to dress the root canal for a time with disinfecting medicaments

- Confirmation of full length access to the root canal can be confirmed using an apex locator or by taking a periapical radiograph with a file inserted to a known length

- To root fill the canal, it is dried and then a gutta percha point smeared with a sealant material is inserted to the previously determined full working length of the root canal

- Similar points are inserted laterally to fully obliterate the full length and width of the root canal (obturation)

- This ensures that no spaces remain for microorganisms to linger and recontaminate the root canal in the future

- The tooth is restored to full function and aesthetics using one of the permanent restorative filling materials (see **Figure 7.2**)

AFTERCARE OF ROOT-TREATED TEETH

Although teeth that have undergone pulpectomy are now non-vital (dead), they can still be subject to carious attack if a consistently good standard of oral hygiene is not maintained, or if they are exposed to a diet high in sugars or acids. The patient will feel no symptoms of thermal sensitivity or pain in

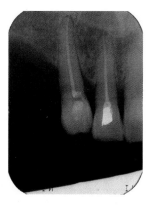

Figure 7.2 Completed root fillings

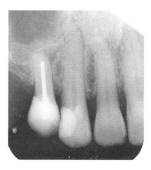

Figure 7.3 Radiograph showing periapical area and metal post in root-filled tooth

these teeth, and only regular dental examinations will detect the presence of any caries.

If left undiagnosed, the root-treated tooth can become so undermined by caries that it fractures, usually catastrophically at the gingival margin of the tooth. It then often requires extensive rebuilding, often involving the insertion of metal or carbon fibre posts into the root canal to anchor and support the rebuilt tooth (see **Figure 7.3**).

If the tooth is unrestorable, it will require extraction.

SECTION 8
TOOTH EXTRACTION

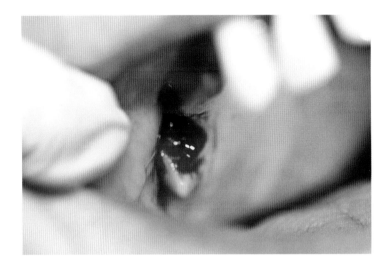

REASON FOR PROCEDURE

Despite the best efforts of the dentist, there are times when a tooth is beyond restoration and has to be extracted. Often, in these circumstances, the patient could suffer from dental infection and pain if the tooth was allowed to remain. The cause of the infection or pain may be gross caries, severe trauma, periodontal disease or failure of an endodontic technique.

There are also several reasons why a tooth may be extracted electively, and these include the following:

- Prosthetic reasons, when the tooth is malaligned and prevents the placement of a denture or bridge

- Severe malalignment that cannot be corrected orthodontically

- To create space in a crowded dental arch so that other teeth can be aligned orthodontically

- Partially erupted and impacted teeth that cannot be cleaned adequately by the patient and suffer from repeated localised infection

- Retained deciduous teeth that prevent their adult successors from erupting correctly

- Patient choice, where the alternative is complicated and possibly expensive dental treatment

In most cases, a tooth can be simply extracted by loosening it in the bony socket and removing it whole, but, in more difficult cases, a surgical procedure may be required.

SIMPLE EXTRACTIONS

Background information of procedure

A tooth is extracted by loosening it in its socket, and then pushing it out of the socket using a variety of dental extraction forceps, elevators or luxators. To loosen the tooth, there must be access to the top of the root or roots for the dentist to hold onto with the extraction forceps – the tooth

TOOTH EXTRACTION

is never held by its crown as this would simply fracture during the procedure.

Alternatively, luxators can be used to sever the periodontal ligament attachment to the tooth and also widen the bony socket so that the tooth is loosened. It is then pushed out of the socket as the instrument is pushed apically.

In successful tooth extraction, physical strength is less of an issue than the skill of the loosening technique used by the dentist.

Details of procedure

No matter how loose a tooth, local anaesthetic should always be administered before an extraction procedure. This must be sufficient to numb not just the tooth, but all of the surrounding gingiva, if the procedure is to be painless for the patient.

The dental nurse maintains good moisture control in the oral cavity using high-speed suction, as well as providing head support to stabilise the patient and assist the dentist during the procedure.

Technique

- A current radiograph of the tooth should be on display so that the dentist is aware of any root curvatures

- The dentist, nurse and patient wear personal protective equipment

- Local anaesthetic is administered and allowed to take full effect

- The dental chair is angled so that the dentist can apply suitable pressure to the tooth without straining, as tooth extraction requires some physical exertion

- The dental nurse firmly but comfortably supports the patient's head to prevent rocking movements, as these will waste the physical effort of the dentist

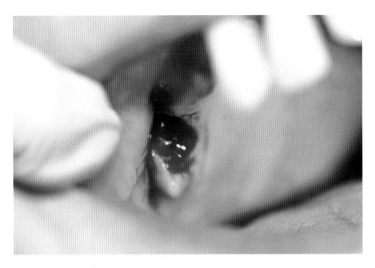

Figure 8.1 Extraction socket

• The dentist uses extraction forceps, luxators and/or elevators to gradually loosen the periodontal attachment of the tooth root to the bony socket walls

• High-speed suction is used by the dental nurse to remove any blood and to keep the operative field visually clear for the dentist

• The tooth is firmly held by the forceps and removed from the oral cavity as the extraction is completed

• A bite pack is placed over the socket and the patient is instructed to bite down hard onto it to achieve haemostasis

• The tooth is inspected to ensure that it has been extracted whole, and that no fractured root fragments remain in the socket

• The socket is inspected once bleeding has stopped to ensure that no bony socket fractures have occurred – any loose sequestrae are removed (see **Figure 8.1**)

- Full verbal and written post-operative instructions are given to the patient to ensure that the socket heals uneventfully

SURGICAL EXTRACTIONS

Background information of procedure

When a tooth has decayed such that caries extends into the root, it is likely to fracture during a simple extraction attempt. Similarly, a heavily filled tooth is weak to the forces applied during extraction and may also fracture and disintegrate during the procedure.

Some teeth, especially multirooted posterior ones, have curved roots that make simple extraction difficult, as attempts to elevate them from the socket in one direction often lock the curved roots in place.

Partially erupted teeth (and obviously unerupted ones) are, by definition, not fully through the gingivae, and so access to their roots for extraction purposes is impossible.

In all of these cases, the dentist will resort to some form of surgical technique to extract the tooth involved, ideally without leaving any pieces *in situ*.

Details of procedure

When a simple extraction cannot be performed because of curved roots, the dentist can often simply section the tooth into two or three separate roots (hemisection or trisection, respectively) and elevate each one as a single root, without the need to peel the gingiva from the underlying bone as a full surgical procedure.

In all other cases of surgical extraction, some degree of gingival and, possibly, bone removal will be required, and so local anaesthetic will always be needed. Specialist surgical instruments are employed, and the dental nurse uses high-speed suction and fine surgical tips to maintain moisture control and to provide a clear operative field for the dentist.

Technique

- A current radiograph of the tooth should be on display for the dentist's reference (see **Figure 8.2**)

- The dentist, nurse and patient wear personal protective equipment

- Local anaesthetic is administered and allowed to take full effect

- The dental chair is angled so that the dentist and nurse have clear visibility of the tooth without straining, as surgical extractions can take some time

- The dentist cuts the surrounding gingiva with a scalpel blade and peels it back from the underlying bone using surgical instruments

- The dental nurse retracts the soft tissues and uses high-speed suction to maintain a clear operative field

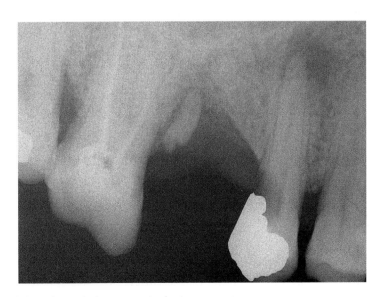

Figure 8.2 Radiograph showing retained root

TOOTH EXTRACTION

TOOTH EXTRACTION

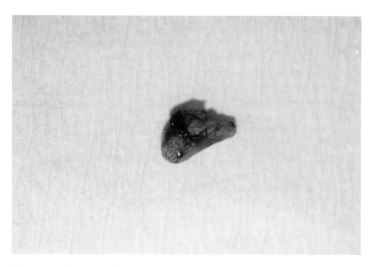

Figure 8.3 Surgically extracted root

- The roots are assessed and bone may be removed to improve access to them, usually using a surgical burr and handpiece with copious irrigation

- Once sufficient bone has been removed, the dentist uses a variety of elevators, luxators and forceps to remove the roots (see **Figure 8.3**)

- Ideally, all the tooth and root pieces are removed, but, occasionally, small but very deeply placed root fragments may remain inaccessible without considerable bone removal

- Decision may be made to leave these *in situ* and to keep under observation radiographically, rather than proceed with excessive bone removal that could weaken the jaw itself

- The patient is informed of this decision at the time

- Once tooth and root removal has been completed, the socket is checked for any loose bony sequestrae, which are removed

- The gingival tissue flap is sutured back into place to cover the underlying bone and to allow healing to occur

- The patient is instructed to clamp onto the bite pack placed over the socket until haemostasis has been achieved

- Full verbal and written post-operative instructions are given to the patient

TOOTH EXTRACTION

TOOTH REPLACEMENT WITH DENTURES

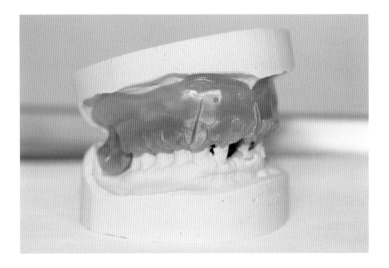

REASON FOR PROCEDURE

Tooth replacement is necessary for several reasons, but mainly to provide adequate masticatory function and to improve aesthetics (see **Figure 9.1**). The absence of one or several teeth may also allow overloading of those remaining, so that excessive tooth wear or even tooth fracture may occur (see **Figure 9.2**). When a tooth is missing, those on either side of it can collapse into the space remaining so that the occlusion is altered, or those in the opposite dental arch can overerupt into the space and cause unnatural wear of the remaining teeth.

Dentures are removable appliances made in several stages in a laboratory, and designed to replace just one or several teeth, or a full dental arch in an edentulous patient (see **Figure 9.3**). Unlike bridges, no tooth preparation is usually required for their construction as long as denture retention is available, and they can be removed from the patient's oral cavity for cleaning as necessary.

They are retained in the mouth by a film of saliva between the oral soft tissues and the denture surface, which provides suction, as well as by the muscular support of the cheeks, lips and tongue. When the patient has some

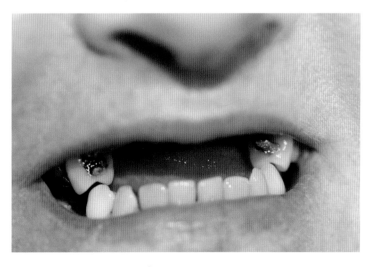

Figure 9.1 Missing upper anterior teeth

TOOTH REPLACEMENT WITH DENTURES

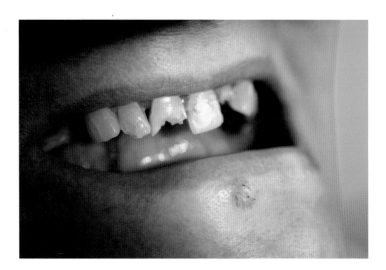

Figure 9.2 Tooth wear with bruxism

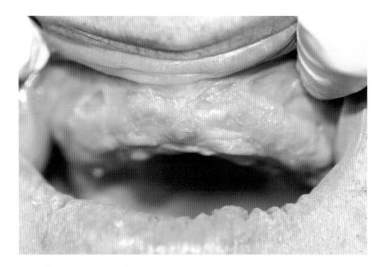

Figure 9.3 Edentulous upper ridge

of his or her own teeth present, additional retention can be provided by using metal clasps incorporated in the denture design to grip these standing teeth.

The base of the denture can be constructed using a pink or transparent acrylic material, or a very thin skeleton design of chrome–cobalt metal. The latter tends to be more comfortable to wear and more hygienic, as less soft tissue is covered, but usually requires the additional retention provided by clasps on suitably positioned standing teeth.

Those to be discussed are:

• Full or partial acrylic dentures

• Full or partial chrome dentures

• Immediate replacement dentures

FULL OR PARTIAL ACRYLIC DENTURES

Background information of procedure

Acrylic dentures are the most common type of denture provided, as they are cheaper and more easily constructed than chrome dentures. They are also more easily adjusted to fit as necessary, as well as being more amenable to relining and tooth addition as the patient's oral cavity alters with time. However, they can fracture during normal usage in patients with heavy bites, or if they are inadvertently dropped whilst out of the mouth.

Nonetheless, acrylic dentures fulfil their necessary function of restoring the patient's occlusion so that adequate mastication is possible, as well as improving appearance, especially when anterior teeth are missing.

Whether one tooth, several teeth or all of the dental arch is to be replaced, the construction procedure for acrylic dentures is basically the same.

Details of procedure

The denture construction normally takes up to five appointments, as each stage must be sent to a laboratory for the next stage to be constructed. When a partial denture is being made, the tooth shade is chosen to match that of the remaining standing teeth; however, when full dentures are being provided, any shade can be chosen, although the dentist will tend to advise a natural creamy shade rather than a more unnatural stark white colour.

Technique

- The dentist, nurse and patient wear personal protective equipment at each appointment

- The dental chair is kept upright for patient comfort, as well as to obtain the ideal position for the dentist to access the oral cavity for this procedure

- Initial impressions are taken in alginate material. They are sent to the laboratory for study model casting and for the construction of personalised impression trays and wax bite recording rims (see **Figure 9.4**)

- At the next appointment, accurate impressions are taken in one of the elastomeric impression materials available using the specially constructed

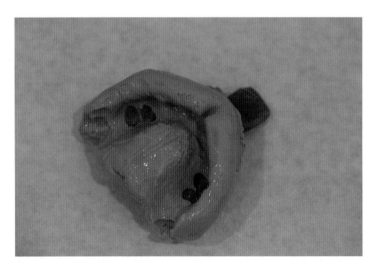

Figure 9.4 Upper alginate impression

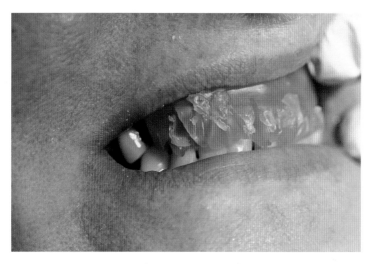

Figure 9.5 Bite record in mouth

impression trays, and the final decision on tooth shade and shape is made by the dentist and the patient

- Occlusal bite recording is carried out using the wax bite rims, so that a partially dentate patient has the same bite with the denture as without, and an edentulous patient can have his or her bite set at a comfortable position to allow speech and mastication, without the jaws being closed up or opened too much (see **Figure 9.5**)

- Wax bite rims will have been warmed and stuck together during the bite recording process and, once placed onto the study models, the technician can reproduce the patient's bite accurately (see **Figure 9.6**)

- In complicated cases, the study models may be mounted onto an articulator at the laboratory

- At the next appointment, a waxed-up try-in of the denture is provided, with the teeth set at the previously recorded occlusion and in the shade and shape chosen (see **Figure 9.7**)

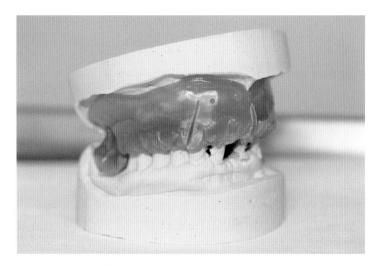

Figure 9.6 Bite rim on model

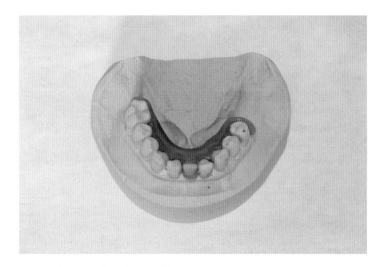

Figure 9.7 Acrylic try-in placed on model

- The fit of the denture is assessed for accuracy, although it will feel slack to the patient as the wax base warms in the mouth

- The occlusion and aesthetics of the denture are assessed, and any minor adjustments can be carried out at the chairside by simply selectively warming the wax bases and adjusting the teeth as necessary

- If any major adjustments are needed, the try-in is returned to the laboratory with details of the adjustments required, and a re-try appointment is arranged

- Once the dentist and patient are happy with the try-in, it is returned to the laboratory, where a flasking process is carried out to replace the wax base with the permanent acrylic material, as the final construction stage of the denture

- If metal clasps are being used for additional retention with a partial denture, they are added at this final stage (see **Figure 9.8**)

- At the final appointment, the completed denture is checked for any sharp edges or specks on the fitting surface before being tried in the patient's mouth, as these would cause soft tissue trauma with time if left

- The denture is then tried in the patient's mouth and assessed for accuracy of fit, function and aesthetics (see **Figure 9.9**)

- Minor occlusal adjustments can be carried out using an acrylic trimming burr and the low-speed handpiece, so that the patient has an even occlusion around the full dental arch

- Post-operative verbal and written care and cleaning instructions are given to the patient

TOOTH REPLACEMENT WITH DENTURES

FULL OR PARTIAL CHROME DENTURES

Background information of procedure

Chrome dentures provide a strong alternative to acrylic in patients with such a heavy bite that they continually fracture their denture base. As chrome can also be constructed as a relatively thin base relative to acrylic, it is the material of choice in patients who gag easily whilst wearing dentures.

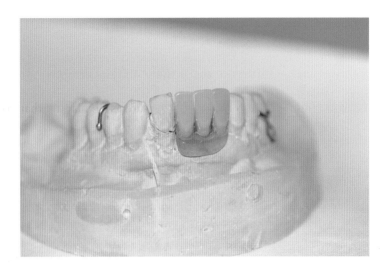

Figure 9.8 Lower partial acrylic denture at fit stage, on model

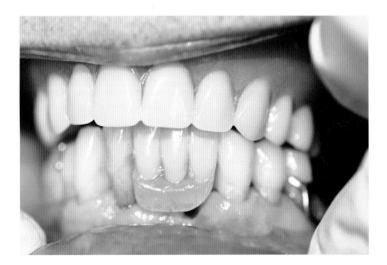

Figure 9.9 Acrylic dentures in place

As the chrome is so strong, the denture can be designed to have minimal soft tissue coverage and not to cover the gingival margins of the teeth, where plaque accumulates so easily. Consequently, chrome dentures are far more hygienic for the patient, and more tissue-friendly to the gingivae.

The construction of a chrome partial denture is similar to that for an acrylic one, but is less amenable to any inaccuracies of design and fit, as once the chrome–cobalt base has been cast it cannot be added to or adjusted.

Details of procedure

The denture construction normally takes up to five appointments, with each stage being sent to a laboratory, as with acrylic dentures. Second impressions must be taken using the special trays made from the study models, as these must be accurate for the chrome base to be constructed well and to fit correctly.

Technique

- The dentist, nurse and patient wear personal protective equipment for each appointment

- The dental chair is kept upright for patient comfort and for ease of access for the dentist

- Initial impressions are taken in alginate material. They are sent to the laboratory for the casting of study models and for the construction of special impression trays and wax bite recording rims

- In partially dentate patients, the denture design is developed to make use of all naturally retentive features by placing clasps on suitable undercut teeth

- At the next appointment, accurate impressions are taken in the special trays using one of the many elastomeric impression materials available, such as silicone or polyether

- Occlusal bite recording is carried out using the wax rims, either to maintain the same occlusion or to adjust it accordingly for an edentulous patient

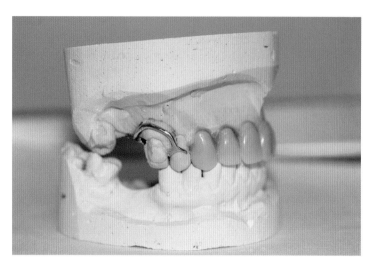

Figure 9.10 Partial chrome try-in on model

- Again, these can be mounted on an articulator in the laboratory by the technician, if necessary

- The final decision on shade and tooth shape is made by the dentist and the patient

- At the next appointment, the chrome–cobalt base design, including all clasps, is available to try in the patient's mouth for accuracy of fit and design (see **Figure 9.10**)

- Any discrepancies in the metal base will require a re-casting to be carried out by the laboratory

- The teeth may also have been added at this stage for a wax try-in, or may be added as an additional stage once the metal work has been approved (see **Figure 9.11**)

- The occlusion and aesthetics of the denture are assessed once the tooth try-in is received, and any minor adjustments are corrected at the chairside

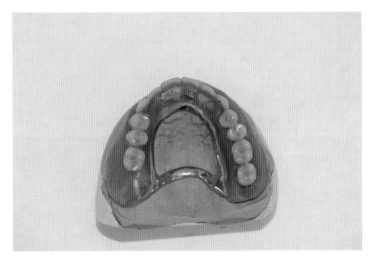

Figure 9.11 Chrome and tooth try-in placed on model

- Once the dentist and patient are happy with both the metal and tooth try-in, it is returned to the laboratory for the flasking process to join the metal base to the acrylic gingivae and teeth (see **Figure 9.12**)

- At the final appointment, the completed denture is checked once again for accuracy of fit, function and aesthetics (see **Figures 9.13 & 9.14**)

- Minor occlusal adjustments can be carried out using an acrylic trimming burr and the low-speed handpiece, but the metal base should require no adjustments

- Post-operative verbal and written care and cleaning instructions are given to the patient

IMMEDIATE REPLACEMENT DENTURES

Background information of procedure

As their name suggests, immediate replacement dentures are those that are fitted at the same time as one or several teeth are extracted. They are usually

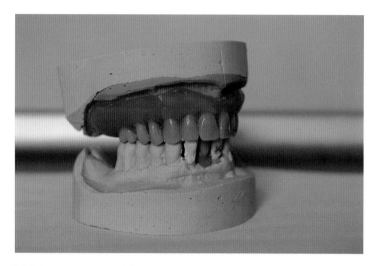

Figure 9.12 Try-in set onto model

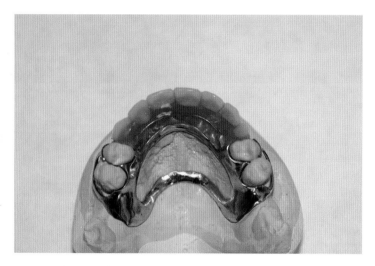

Figure 9.13 Partial chrome fit on model

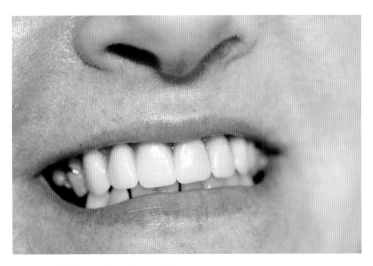

Figure 9.14 Partial chrome fit in the mouth

provided when a patient is to lose one or several anterior teeth and requires the extracted teeth to be replaced at the same time for aesthetic reasons, rather than have visible unsightly spaces for a while.

Although the aesthetic concerns of the patient are very understandable in these circumstances, it must be accepted that the resulting denture will not be as accurate a fit as if it had been constructed conventionally – after tooth extraction.

As a result of the usual event of bone resorption occurring after extraction, the denture will also become slack relatively quickly and will require relining or even remaking at some point.

As these alterations are expected to be required, the immediate replacement denture is always made from acrylic, which can be quite easily added to and adjusted.

When significant bone resorption has finished, usually after 4–6 months, a new denture can be constructed in chrome–cobalt if required.

Details of procedure

The appliance construction follows similar stages to that of a conventional denture, except that there may be no possibility or requirement for a try-in if no other teeth are missing except those to be immediately replaced by the denture (see **Figure 9.15**).

It is imperative that the completed denture is ready for fitting on the day on which the patient is due to have the extractions carried out.

Technique

- The dentist, nurse and patient wear personal protective equipment for each appointment

- The dental chair is kept upright for patient comfort and ease of access for the dentist

- Initial impressions are taken in alginate material, and are sent to the laboratory for study model casting and, possibly, for special tray construction

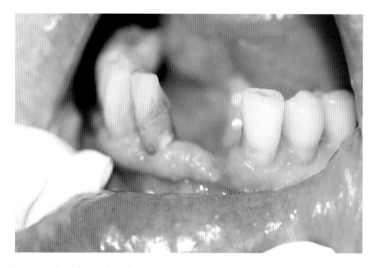

Figure 9.15 Teeth to be replaced

- A special tray may not be necessary if only one tooth is to be replaced immediately, as the completed denture is expected to be less accurate than a conventional one

- Similarly, wax bite rims may also not be necessary if the study models can easily be placed into the correct occlusion without them

- In these simple one-tooth cases, it is usual to take a shade at the initial impression stage and proceed directly to the final acrylic construction of the denture

- Otherwise, the second accurate impression and occlusal bite recording are carried out at the next appointment, as usual

- The final decision on tooth shade is made by the dentist and the patient, and the technician copies the tooth shapes from the study models

- At the next appointment, a waxed try-in of any teeth already missing is provided, but of course the teeth to be immediately replaced cannot be present at this stage

- The try-in is checked for accuracy of fit, occlusion and aesthetics as far as possible, and any minor adjustments are carried out at the chairside

- Once the try-in and study models are returned to the laboratory for completion of the denture, the technician carefully removes the teeth to be extracted from the model and replaces them with suitable denture teeth, ensuring that the occlusion is not altered during the process

- The flasking process is carried out to replace the wax base with the permanent acrylic of the denture (see **Figure 9.16**)

- At the final appointment, the teeth to be replaced are extracted under local anaesthetic and, once haemostasis has been achieved, the denture is inserted into the patient's mouth

- The aesthetics are checked, and the fit and occlusion are examined as far as possible bearing in mind that the patient will still be numb from the local anaesthetic

- Post-operative verbal and written care and cleaning instructions are given to the patient, and a review appointment is provisionally made so that any

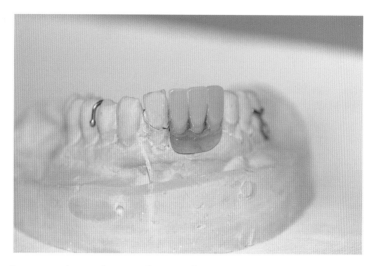

Figure 9.16 Immediate replacement denture at fit stage

problems that become apparent once the local anaesthetic has worn off can be corrected

AFTERCARE OF DENTURES

Any type of denture is designed to be a removable appliance, one that the patient can take out of the mouth for cleaning purposes and leave out overnight. Acrylic partial dentures are designed to fit around any standing teeth, and these areas will allow plaque to accumulate and cause either localised caries of standing teeth or periodontal disease if the plaque is not removed promptly.

As chrome dentures are usually designed to cover less oral soft tissue, they tend not to allow such plaque accumulations to develop. Plaque is still produced in patients with no natural teeth of their own and, if left on the fitting surface of any full denture being worn, will provide ideal conditions for fungal development and infection with oral thrush.

Dentures should be cleaned at least twice daily using either a specific denture paste or ordinary toothpaste with a toothbrush. They are best cleaned over a bowl of water to avoid breakages if dropped, and should be rinsed well before reinserting.

Various denture soaking agents are available for use overnight; however, care should be taken with bleach-based ones as these are not suitable for chrome dentures and cause metal corrosion with time.

SECTION 10

TOOTH REPLACEMENT WITH IMPLANTS

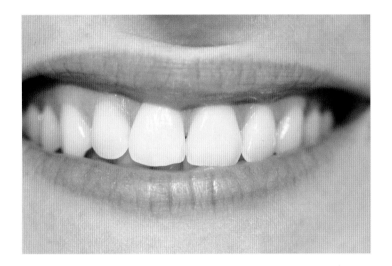

REASON FOR PROCEDURE

Missing teeth can be replaced using bridges, dentures or implants. Each technique has its own advantages and disadvantages, but they are all required for the same reasons – to provide adequate masticatory function and to improve aesthetics.

Implants are the most advanced technique of tooth replacement, although their use has been developing over at least the last 30 years. They involve the surgical placement of a threaded titanium cylinder (implant) into the jaw bone, which then has an abutment screwed into its top end to project into the oral cavity. This abutment then forms the attachment for a crown replacing a single tooth, a bridge retainer replacing several teeth or an overdenture replacing many, if not all, of the teeth in a dental arch.

The advantage of implants over other methods of tooth replacement is that they can be used in patients without having to cut into adjacent teeth to construct bridgework and in patients with very poor retention for conventional dentures.

However, these more complicated cases can involve all of the following:

- An oral and/or periodontal surgeon

- A specialist in prosthetics

- Advanced computerised radiographic techniques

- A specialist implant laboratory

The procedure described is for the simpler replacement of a single tooth only.

SINGLE TOOTH IMPLANTS

Background information of procedure

Even when a single tooth is to be replaced, a detailed dental and radiographic assessment of the patient must be carried out by the dentist beforehand. This will determine the feasibility of placing the implant and its likelihood of success, as well as the suitability of the patient for the procedure and his or her likelihood of complying with the long-term care of the restoration.

The initial placement of the implant cylinder is a full surgical technique, and is usually left *in situ* for up to 6 months whilst the jaw bone grows around it to anchor it firmly. Only then is the abutment attached and the single tooth crown constructed and placed.

During the interim period, the patient must be provided with either a temporary denture or a temporary etch retained bridge to replace the missing tooth and to sit comfortably over the implant head.

However, more recently, a technique has been developed whereby the implant cylinder is placed at the time of tooth extraction, and a single crown is fitted over the top. This can only be performed when the replaced tooth is kept free from occlusal loading, so that the bony attachment between implant and jaw bone can occur.

Details of procedure

Only dentists who have been suitably trained to provide implants can undertake the procedure, as the technique is a specialised field that is not covered by undergraduate training.

In a normal situation, the patient will have an anterior tooth missing and replaced either by a denture or an acid etch retained bridge. The latter will need to be removed intact before the implant placement, and then adjusted as necessary and re-attached whilst the healing process occurs. All necessary radiographs and study models must be taken and assessed beforehand.

Specialist surgical instruments and equipment are required, and the dental nurse must maintain good moisture control throughout the procedure.

Technique

- Current radiographs of the implant site should be available for reference by the dentist, and the implant dimensions and required angulation of insertion must be determined beforehand

- The dentist, nurse and patient wear personal protective equipment at each appointment

- The dental chair is placed at an angle to allow easy and comfortable access for the dentist and nurse, as well as full visibility of the operative site

- Local anaesthetic is administered to all the surrounding oral soft tissues and allowed to take full effect

- The dentist cuts the surrounding gingiva with a scalpel blade and peels it back from the underlying bone using surgical instruments

- The dental nurse retracts the soft tissues and uses high-speed suction to maintain a clear operative field, and provides copious irrigation during bone surgery

- The jaw bone ridge is flattened at the point at which the implant is to be inserted

- A hole is drilled into the jaw bone at the correct angulation and depth using specialist implant drills (mill)

- The prepared depth is checked using a calibrated depth gauge

- The chosen implant is driven into the jaw bone using specialist insert instruments and a surgical hammer

- The gingival tissue flaps are repositioned to close the surgical site, with just the implant head projecting through

- The head is covered with a plastic cap, and a temporary denture or temporary etch retained bridge is replaced whilst healing occurs

- Full verbal and written post-operative instructions are given to the patient

- Following 3 months of healing and attachment of the implant to the surrounding jaw bone, the plastic cap is removed and a suitable abutment is screwed into the implant cylinder

- Its shape is that of a conventionally prepared crown core, and its size is dictated by the adjacent tooth positions and the patient's occlusion

- An accurate impression is taken of the abutment and adjacent teeth using a silicone or polyether elastomeric material, and opposing arch impression and occlusion are recorded in the usual way

- The technician constructs the crown in the laboratory using the same procedure as for a conventional crown

- At the final appointment, the crown is cemented onto the abutment after checking for fit, function and aesthetics

- Full verbal and written post-operative instructions are given to the patient

AFTERCARE OF IMPLANTS

Although the implant cannot be affected by caries, it can develop plaque accumulations around it and allow a periodontal infection to occur. Ultimately, this can result in the formation of periodontal pockets around the implant, destruction of the bone–implant attachment and loosening of the implant itself.

As with real teeth, the prevention of periodontal infection depends on the use of a consistently high standard of oral hygiene by the patient. This should include correct toothbrushing, the use of interdental cleaning aids around the implant and the use of a good quality toothpaste and mouthwash.

Regular dental examinations should be carried out on both the real teeth and the implant, and regular oral hygiene reinforcement and scaling should be performed as necessary.

TOOTH REPLACEMENT WITH IMPLANTS

SECTION 11

TOOTH ALIGNMENT WITH ORTHODONTIC BRACES

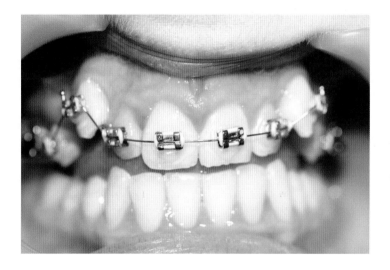

REASON FOR PROCEDURE

Although a patient's desire for straight teeth is usually based on aesthetics, there are several dental advantages to aligning uneven teeth. Crooked and crowded teeth provide many potential areas for plaque to accumulate that would not exist if the dental arch was well aligned (see **Figure 11.1**). It will take a consistently high standard of oral hygiene for life in these cases to prevent any carious or periodontal damage from occurring with time, as each crooked tooth and crowded area will require individual attention during every toothbrushing session.

When teeth are severely crowded, they sometimes do not bite together sufficiently well for the patient to chew food efficiently, and, in very severe cases, where the jaw sizes do not match, the patient may also experience speech difficulties. These severe cases often benefit from a combined approach of orthodontics and jaw surgery.

TOOTH ALIGNMENT WITH
ORTHODONTIC BRACES

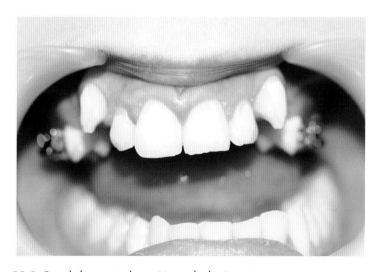

Figure 11.1 Crowded upper teeth requiring orthodontic treatment

When the bottom jaw bites too far behind its normal position, the upper anterior teeth will appear to project forwards quite prominently (proclined), and these upper teeth will be vulnerable to trauma or even fracture by being so positioned.

Finally, the psychological well-being of a patient should be considered in severe cases, when malocclusion may be responsible for excessively low self-esteem or the cause of childhood teasing or even bullying.

The simplest techniques used for tooth alignment are:

• Removable appliances

• Fixed appliances

REMOVABLE APPLIANCES

Background information of procedure

Removable appliances are made from an acrylic base with metal attachments to provide retention, similar to acrylic dentures. They have additional metal components incorporated as necessary to carry out the required tooth movement to be achieved, and these include a variety of springs, screw devices or adjustable metal bars.

These components are checked and adjusted by the dentist on a regular basis to effect the tooth movement.

When severe crowding is present in the dental arch, it may be necessary for tooth extraction to be carried out before an appliance is fitted. This creates the space required to reposition the other teeth and align the arch.

The amount of movement possible with a removable appliance is sufficient in many cases to fully correct malaligned teeth, but the force applied is limited by the fact that the appliance is removable – if too much force is applied, the brace is not stable in the mouth. It is then that a fixed appliance is required.

Whichever type of appliance is planned, many new plaque retention areas will be created in the patient's oral cavity, and it is imperative that a consistently good standard of oral hygiene and diet control is practised throughout the course of orthodontic treatment.

Poor oral hygiene is the main factor preventing many patients from being offered orthodontic treatment, no matter how great their need.

Details of procedure

The dentist carries out an oral and radiographic assessment of the patient beforehand, and determines the orthodontic treatment required and the appliance necessary to achieve it by taking study model impressions and studying the casts produced. The need for any tooth extractions is decided, and the full treatment course is explained to the patient to determine his or her willingness to undergo orthodontic treatment. This includes the requirement for the appliance to be worn at all times, except for meals, and the need for good diet control and oral hygiene throughout the full course of treatment.

If amenable, the removable appliance can be constructed.

Technique

- The dentist, nurse and patient wear personal protective equipment at each appointment

- Alginate impressions are taken of both dental arches to produce the working casts for the technician

- A written design of the appliance is sent with the impressions

- The patient receives oral hygiene instruction and dietary advice

- At the next appointment, the new appliance is checked for accuracy of design and then tried in the patient's mouth (see **Figure 11.2**)

- Once comfortably tight, any metal components involved in tooth movement are activated by the dentist, and the treatment commences (see **Figure 11.3**)

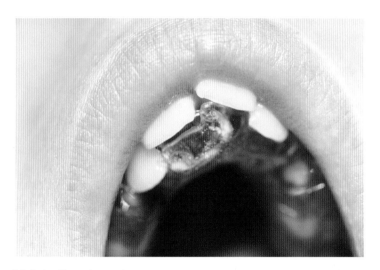

Figure 11.2 Appliance in mouth

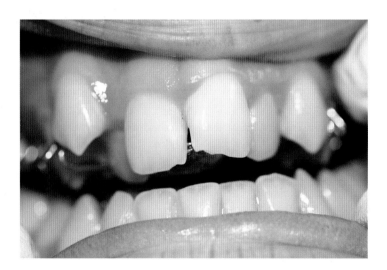

Figure 11.3 Active spring on central incisor

- Specific oral hygiene instruction is given for the appliance itself, as well as the wearing details

- At each appointment thereafter, the dentist checks the progress of the tooth movement against the original study casts to ensure that it is progressing correctly

- Retentive cribs are tightened to ensure that the appliance is not loose, and active components are adjusted accordingly

- Once the tooth movement required has been achieved, a retainer may be provided to hold the teeth in their new positions until they have settled into alignment

- A retainer can be either the deactivated removable appliance itself or a soft gum shield type, both of which are worn at night only

FIXED APPLIANCES

Background information of procedure

As their name suggests, fixed appliances are actually bonded onto the patient's teeth for the duration of the orthodontic treatment. In this way, greater forces can be applied and more severely malaligned teeth can be corrected than can be achieved with removable appliances alone.

However, greater care is needed by the patient during normal day-to-day activities so as not to dislodge any components of the appliance, as it cannot be removed for meals, cleaning or during sport sessions, as can a removable appliance. Similarly, a low-sugar/low-acid diet must be strictly followed, as the number of plaque retentive areas created by a fixed appliance is huge, and caries can easily occur.

The fixed appliance consists of individual metal brackets and bands that are harmlessly bonded onto each tooth in exactly the correct position, and then all joined together by fixing a continuous archwire into each component. The wire carefully guides the movement of each tooth along it, gradually aligning the dental arch as it does so. The wire is changed on a regular basis

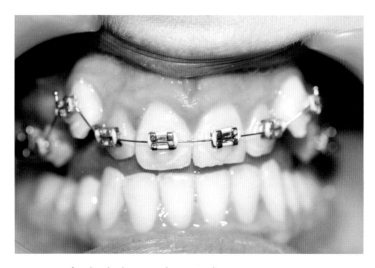

Figure 11.4 Upper fixed orthodontic appliance in place

by the dentist, using thicker, less flexible wires as the treatment progresses (see **Figure 11.4**).

As with removable appliances, tooth extraction may be required first to create space in the dental arch.

Details of procedure

The dentist carries out an oral and radiographic assessment of the patient beforehand, and determines the order and progression of the archwires required using the initial study casts. The need for any tooth extraction is decided upon and discussed with the patient when presenting the treatment plan. The strict diet and oral hygiene control are also explained, and the patient can then decide if he or she is willing to proceed with the full course of orthodontic treatment. If amenable, the fixed appliance can be fitted.

Technique

- The dentist, nurse and patient wear personal protective equipment at each appointment

- The dental chair is placed supine for ease of access, and good moisture control is provided throughout the bonding appointment using low-speed suction and cotton wool rolls

- A decision will have been made previously with regard to whether one or both dental arches are to be bonded at the same appointment

- The teeth are blown dry and a spot of acid etch is applied to the centre of the labial surface of each tooth in the dental arch

- The etch is washed off and carefully collected using high-speed suction, and then the teeth are dried again

- The individual brackets are then bonded, one at a time, in exactly the correct position and at the correct angulation for each tooth, using a special orthodontic material similar to composite

- Any bands required are sized on the tooth and then cemented firmly into place using any material that is employed for crown cementation

- Once all the tooth attachments are firmly in place, the first archwire is positioned and tied onto each attachment using special elastic loops

- The first archwire is usually the thinnest and most flexible available, as it needs to be accurately distorted into each attachment, no matter how malaligned the teeth sit in the dental arch

- The archwire ends are trimmed to avoid sticking into the patient's cheeks

- Detailed oral hygiene instructions are given for the thorough cleaning of the appliance, without dislodging it

- At each appointment thereafter, progress is checked against the original study casts to ensure that the required tooth movement is proceeding correctly

- The archwire is replaced as necessary with a gradually thicker and less flexible successor as the dental arch gradually aligns

- Once the tooth movement required has been achieved, a retainer is constructed for each dental arch to hold the teeth in their new positions until they have settled into alignment

- The retainer may be a soft gum shield type, to be worn at night only, or a fixed wire bonded to the backs of the teeth for a firmer method of retention

AFTERCARE OF ORTHODONTIC BRACES

As with acrylic dentures, removable appliances are cleaned with a toothbrush and fluoride toothpaste over a bowl of water after each meal. This is especially important at bedtime as the orthodontic appliance must be worn overnight. The patient must also clean his or her own teeth thoroughly after each meal whilst the appliance is out, in the usual manner.

Fixed appliances must be thoroughly cleaned *in situ* after each meal using a combination of toothbrush, fluoride toothpaste and interdental brushes employed specifically to clean beneath the archwire itself.

Some good quality electric toothbrushes have special orthodontic heads for use by the patient during the course of orthodontic treatment.

Patients with removable appliances are advised to store the brace in a rigid container whilst out of the mouth at mealtimes or during sport sessions, to avoid breakages. Fixed appliances can be protected from damage during sport sessions using specially designed shields that fit over them in the mouth. These will also prevent soft tissue trauma if the patient inadvertently receives a blow to the mouth; however, contact sports are best avoided during the course of orthodontic treatment.

If oral hygiene is not sufficiently maintained, or the diet not correctly controlled, the patient risks developing caries in any tooth, but especially in teeth that are in contact with the orthodontic appliance. In fixed appliance cases, this can result in unsightly cavities on the most visible part of each tooth, which will require permanent restorations for life.

SECTION 12
TOOTH WHITENING

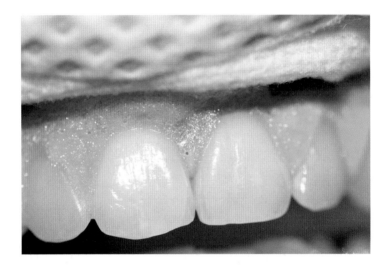

REASON FOR PROCEDURE

In an increasingly appearance-conscious society, tooth whitening is becoming a more popular treatment for patients. In the majority of cases, it is carried out for aesthetic reasons only; however, some patients have unnaturally dark teeth that cause great embarrassment and low self-esteem. As with some orthodontic patients, the dentist is in a position to improve the quality of life of these patients by performing a relatively simple and non-invasive technique.

There are a variety of tooth whitening systems available, including over-the-counter products and whitening toothpastes on sale direct to the patient.

When used correctly, they are all perfectly safe and cause no damage to the teeth. The alternative dental treatment to achieve tooth whitening is to undergo multiple veneer or crown preparations, and all of the long-term maintenance and care of these restorations that this entails.

The procedures to be discussed are:

- Home whitening using trays

- In-house power whitening

HOME WHITENING USING TRAYS

Background information of procedure

This is a simple technique whereby the patient self-determines the use of the product and the end result achieved. It involves the use of specially constructed trays – similar to thin gum shields or orthodontic retainers – that are worn at home by the patient with the whitening paste within them. The trays can be worn as little or as often as the patient decides; obviously, greater usage produces a greater whitening effect, but a noticeable improvement in tooth shade normally takes weeks to develop.

As long as the trays fit accurately around the teeth, the treatment course can be repeated as often as the patient wishes. The whitening paste will have no effect on any restorations already present, such as white fillings or crowns,

TOOTH WHITENING

and so these may require replacement at a later date if the shade difference is noticeable.

Details of procedure

Several home whitening products are available to the dental profession, but all rely on the use of custom-made trays to hold the paste on the surfaces of the teeth for long enough to have an effect. Other than provision of the product and construction of the trays for each patient, the dentist has little input to the procedure.

Technique

- The dentist, nurse and patient wear personal protective equipment

- Alginate impressions are taken of one or both dental arches for the working models to be cast

- Using a shade guide provided by the whitening paste manufacturers, the patient's tooth shade is recorded so that the degree of whitening achieved can be quantified

- A photograph may also be taken and kept in the patient's record card for future reference

- Cast models are used to construct the customised, vacuum formed trays for each patient, either in-house or at a laboratory

- At the next appointment, the trays are checked for accuracy of fit and the paste application into the tray is demonstrated to the patient

- Excessive amounts of paste should not be used, as this is not only wasteful but the excess will spill onto the soft tissues and may cause irritation

- Each consignment of whitening paste has patient information details enclosed, and these are explained verbally and then given to the patient for home reference

- The patient can request more whitening paste as necessary

IN-HOUSE POWER WHITENING

Background information of procedure

As the name suggests, this is a whitening technique that provides an instant result for the patient after just one application. It relies on the use of an intense light source to chemically activate the whitening process of the paste after it has been applied to the teeth, and must be performed in a controlled environment at the practice.

As the activated paste is so intense, all of the soft tissues of the oral cavity must be protected from contact with it during the procedure to avoid soft tissue irritation or burns. Similarly, the patient's face and lips should be protected from the light source by covering with total block suncream and lip balm.

Details of procedure

Suitable patients should be chosen carefully, as the intense nature of the procedure can cause temporary tooth sensitivity, which is sometimes intense in nature. In addition, some medications and even herbal products can cause the patient to be oversensitive to the light source used, resulting in sunburn or sunstroke-like symptoms. Careful pre-operative questioning will identify any likely problems.

The shade guide is used to determine the pre-treatment tooth shade, and may be photographically recorded.

Technique

- The dentist, nurse and patient wear personal protective equipment throughout the procedure, especially orange-tinted safety glasses whenever the light source is in use

- The patient is made comfortable in the dental chair, angled at 45°, as the procedure can take up to 2 h once started

- Suncream and lip balm are spread liberally over the patient's facial soft tissues

TOOTH WHITENING

- A special lip and tongue retractor is carefully placed in the mouth so that all oral soft tissues are held away from the teeth

- The inner sides of the lips and cheeks and the surface of the tongue are fully covered with cotton gauze to give full protection and moisture control

- Protective paste is carefully run across all exposed gingival tissues up to the necks of the teeth, and then set hard so that it provides a light-proof barrier for the underlying tissues (see **Figure 12.1**)

- Whitening paste is mixed and carefully applied to the labial surfaces of all anterior teeth

- A power light is positioned directly over the teeth and locked in position for each of the three 15 min cycles of exposure required

- The teeth are washed, dried and fresh whitening paste is reapplied before each exposure

- At the end of the procedure, the new tooth shade is recorded, and the soft tissues are checked for any signs of irritation; a soothing balm is placed if necessary

- The patient is given full post-operative instructions with regard to avoiding smoking and highly coloured foods and drinks for 48 h to prevent staining of the teeth, as the teeth are very porous during this initial period (see **Figure 12.2**)

- Any tooth sensitivity is temporarily and easily alleviated using a desensitising gel provided in each whitening kit

AFTERCARE OF WHITENED TEETH

Any restorations previously present may need replacement, especially with the power whitening technique. Some patients may choose to continue the initial shade improvement achieved with the in-house procedure by using customised trays and home whitening pastes, as described previously.

The period of time over which the whitening effect lasts with no further treatment will depend on the smoking and dietary habits of the patient. In

TOOTH WHITENING

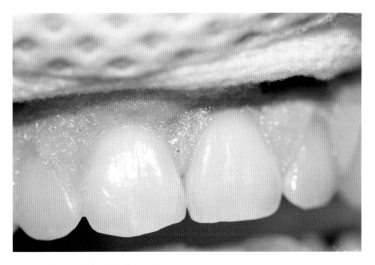

Figure 12.1 Isolation of teeth before whitening

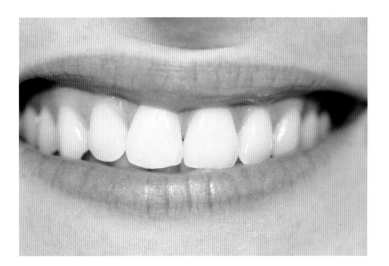

Figure 12.2 End result after power whitening of upper teeth

particular, tea, coffee and red wine are all notorious for causing tooth staining, and advice should be given on reducing their consumption for a lasting
effect after whitening.

As any tooth whitening technique is non-invasive, no special care or maintenance instructions are necessary, except to carry out a good daily oral
hygiene programme.

TOOTH WHITENING

GLOSSARY OF TERMS

Abrasion cavity – a self-inflicted worn area produced at the neck of a tooth by overvigorous toothbrushing

Acid etch – an acidic material used in dentistry on the enamel of a tooth to chemically roughen it, allowing greater adhesion of certain fillings and cements

Acute infection – an infection of sudden onset, and therefore associated with pain and swelling

Aesthetics – relating to a pleasing appearance, as in the aesthetics of a veneer for instance

Apex locator – an electronic device used during root treatment to determine the full length of a root canal by giving off a signal when the apex has been located

Articulating paper – thin carbon paper used to detect high spots on new restorations by being placed between the teeth and leaving coloured marks when the patient occludes

Articulator – a three-dimensional jig device that mimics occlusion and jaw movements when a set of study casts is accurately placed within

Bitewing radiograph – a posterior intra-oral radiographic view taken to show interdental caries or restoration overhangs

Bone resorption – the natural process that occurs in the jaw bones after tooth extraction, so that a smooth ridge contour is produced

Bruxism – the habitual clenching and grinding of the teeth, often causing excessive tooth wear or tooth fracture

Calculus – mineralised deposits of plaque that form at the gingival margins and cause inflammation; it is also referred to as tartar

Caries – a bacterial infection of the hard tissues of the teeth causing cavities; it is also referred to as tooth decay in lay terms

Chronic infection – an infection of very slow but persistent onset, and therefore usually painless

Demineralisation – the action of acids on the tooth enamel to produce weakened areas that are more prone to carious attack

Dentine – the inner living tissue forming the bulk of the tooth structure; it contains nerve endings and therefore allows sensation in the tooth

Edentulous – the condition of having no natural teeth present

Enamel – the outer surface of the erupted crown of a tooth; it is a mineralised, non-living tissue

Fissure – a natural anatomical cleft in the occlusal surface of a tooth between the cusps

Gingival crevice – a 2 mm deep crevice around the necks of all healthy teeth, in which plaque accumulates when oral hygiene standards are poor

Gingival margin – the edge of a restoration (such as a crown) that lies at the gingival crevice

Gingivitis – inflammation of the gingivae, or gums

Gutta percha point – a natural rubber material used to root fill a tooth, and provided in various length and diameter points

Haemostasis – the arrest of blood flow in an area, especially after tooth extraction

Intensifying screen – a device used within extra-oral radiographic cassettes to reduce X-ray exposure to the patient

Interdental area – the area at the point at which two adjacent teeth touch together

Intra-oral radiograph – a radiograph that is exposed to X-rays whilst within the patient's mouth

Labial surface – the outer surface of an anterior tooth that lies against the lips

Lingual surface – the inner surface of any lower tooth that lies against the tongue

Lining – a material used in the base of a cavity before filling to protect the underlying pulp tissue

Luting cement – a cement mixed to a creamy consistency and used as an adhesive in crown and bridge cases

Malalignment – the uneven, out-of-line positions of teeth in a dental arch, often caused by crowding

Mastication – the correct term for the act of the chewing of food

Matrix band – a thin strip of metal or acetate used in a holder to separate adjacent teeth during filling

Moisture control – the act of removing fluid contamination from the oral cavity during dental procedures, often involving the use of suction equipment and absorbent materials

Non-vital tooth – a tooth that has died

Occlusal surface – the biting surface of a posterior tooth

Occlusion – the tooth positions achieved when the jaws are closed together and the upper and lower teeth are contacting

Orthopantomograph – an extra-oral radiograph taken in a cassette, showing the whole of both jaws and their surrounding anatomy

Overdenture – a denture constructed to attach to and fit over the top of implant abutments

Periapical radiograph – an anterior or posterior radiographic view taken to show a full tooth, including its root and the bone immediately surrounding it

Periodontal disease – an infection of the supporting structures of a tooth in its socket by one of several bacterial microorganisms

Periodontal ligament – the tough connective tissue that holds a tooth in its socket

Plaque – a sticky film of food debris and bacteria that forms on the teeth causing caries and gingivitis if not removed

Pulp chamber – the inner hollow chamber of a tooth containing nerve tissue and blood vessels (pulp)

Pulp exposure – the breaching of the pulp chamber and exposure of its contents to the oral cavity

Refined sugar – a sugar not naturally present in a food but added during manufacture, and highly cariogenic

Root apex – the very tip of a tooth root where nerves and blood vessels enter and leave the tooth

Rubber dam – a sheet of rubbery material used to isolate a tooth during dental procedures to provide good moisture control

Saliva – the watery fluid naturally produced by the salivary glands and emptied into the oral cavity to provide lubrication, amongst other functions

Scaler – an instrument used to remove calculus from teeth and roots

Stagnation area – any area in the oral cavity that allows the accumulation of plaque to occur, either present naturally, such as the fissures of the teeth, or produced artificially, such as overhanging filling edges

Stock tray – a plastic or metal standard shaped tray used for taking initial impressions or study model casts

Supine – lying horizontally, as in the usual working position of the dental chair during procedures such as restorations

Vasoconstrictor – a chemical added to local anaesthetic solutions to prolong anaesthesia by constricting the surrounding blood vessels

X-ray cassette – a specialised case containing intensifying screens, used for extra-oral radiography such as orthopantomographs

INDEX

A00000107039323